DOCTORS IN DENIAL

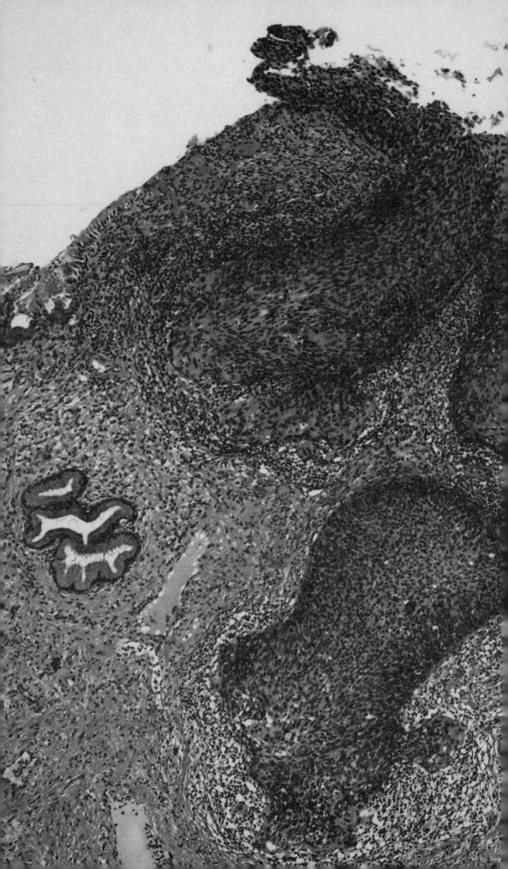

DOCTORS IN DENIAL

The forgotten women in the 'unfortunate experiment'

Ronald W. Jones

OTAGO

Published by Otago University Press
Level 1, 398 Cumberland Street
Dunedin, New Zealand
university.press@otago.ac.nz
www.otago.ac.nz/press

First published 2017
Copyright © Ronald W. Jones

ISBN 978-0-947522-43-8

Cover photograph: Photomicrograph of a section of a cervix, showing carcinoma *in-situ* (front cover) transitioning to invasive cancer (back cover). Courtesy of Drs Sadiq Al Sakini and Mee Ling Yeong

Printed in China through Asia Pacific Offset

CONTENTS

*This book is dedicated to Barbara Jones and Bill McIndoe.
Both battled with cancer. Neither lived to see the outcome
of their endeavours.
It is also dedicated to the women involved in the 'unfortunate experiment'
at National Women's Hospital, Auckland, New Zealand.*

*The years, as they roll by, leave behind them memories that increasingly
pile up until, when 75 years have tolled, they form a large untidy heap
which, if sorted out, would be the history of a life.*

AFTER VICTOR BONNEY, 1952

*All royalties received from the sale of this book will be donated for
gynaecological cancer care and research.*

ACKNOWLEDGEMENTS

I HAVE BEEN EXTRAORDINARILY fortunate to have had a foundation of support from Professor Sir David Skegg, Professors Charlotte Paul and Malcolm Coppleson, and Hugh Rennie QC. Their wisdom, advice, encouragement and willingness to listen have sustained me during this 30-year saga. More recently Professors John Werry, Peter Stone and Dr Bob Gudex have also encouraged me and endorsed my project.

I would also like to acknowledge the interest in my book among my colleagues in the ISSVD, IFCPC and ASCCP. I am particularly appreciative of the support of my friend and colleague Professor Neville Hacker, who wrote the foreword.

This book has been enhanced by vignettes and quotes from many people who have approached me anxious to share their stories. Sadly, a number whose advice I have valued have died during the writing of this book – Professors Sir John Scott and Barbara Heslop, and Drs Bernie Kyle and Ian Ronayne. To all of these colleagues and friends I extend my gratitude.

Over the years I have been blessed with a number of wonderful secretaries who, beyond the call of duty, have typed and retyped endless drafts of my scientific papers and/or early drafts of this book: Glenise Alley, Gail Langley, Jackie Bregman, Diane Ambler, Mark Barrios, Dorothy Burrows – and Sam, who in addition to secretarial responsibilities, has ensured I have not 'given up'.

Librarian Jenny Hobson, artist Diane Stephenson and photographer Jonathan Ellison have generously contributed their skills. The cover of the book displays a photomicrograph kindly provided by Drs Sadiq Al Sakini and Mee Ling Yeong.

A book is not produced by an author alone; when the writing process ends, an editorial and production team take over. I have benefited from the professionalism of Rachel Scott and her team at Otago University Press in bringing this project to completion: I would like to thank them sincerely for their encouragement and patience throughout this process.

RON JONES

FOREWORD

NEVILLE F. HACKER AM

Past President, International Gynecologic Cancer Society

DOCTORS IN DENIAL – the title says it all. Thirty years after the Cartwright Inquiry endorsed the reality of the 'unfortunate experiment', there are still individuals who are denying the truth.

I was completely unaware of the study Associate Professor Herb Green had begun in 1966 into the natural history of carcinoma in-situ (CIS) of the cervix until the long-term results were published in 1984 by Drs William McIndoe, Malcolm McLean and Ronald Jones (with statistician Peter Mullins). Since beginning my training in obstetrics and gynaecology in Brisbane in 1974, I had never heard anyone question the malignant potential of cervical CIS.

Although I was unaware of Green and his work until 1984, I was aware of the incredibly important work emanating from National Women's Hospital in Auckland in the field of perinatology. Professor Bill Liley had performed the world's first intrauterine transfusion for rhesus incompatibility, and Professor Mont Liggins had pioneered work that markedly improved the survival of premature babies. Liley and Liggins were household names in obstetric circles when I began training, and scarcely a labour ward round would go by without reference to their work. I was amazed that two of the most eminent scholars in our field were working at the same hospital, just across the Tasman.

I never met any of the key players in the 'unfortunate experiment', but in this book Professor Ron Jones brings each character to life. Herb Green was a 'tall, balding man with a shambling gait'. He was trusted by his colleagues, and there was a degree of sympathy for him as he had missed out on the postgraduate chair in 1963. He was considered to be a good teacher, but 'held unconventional views' and had an 'uneasy' relationship with his departmental chair, Professor Dennis Bonham. The latter was a 'large, intimidating man', who could easily fly into a rage. His professorial position and difficult character isolated him from many colleagues, but he supported Green whenever there was any challenge to Green's experiment. Bonham tried unsuccessfully to obstruct publication of the 1984 article that exposed the experiment, and was ultimately found guilty of 'disgraceful conduct' by the Medical Council.

Dr William McIndoe was a warm, quietly spoken, meticulous man with strong Christian beliefs. His expertise in colposcopy was used by Green to exclude invasive cancer at the outset. He privately suggested that Green was retrospectively manipulating the data, and withdrew his colposcopic services from Green's study in 1973. Dr Malcolm (Jock) McLean was appointed head pathologist at National Women's in 1961. Somewhat eccentric but unpretentious, he was 'an excellent and much respected teacher' who clashed regularly with Green over the interpretation of cervical pathology. Ron Jones was appointed as a junior gynaecologist at the National Women's Hospital in 1973, seven years after the start of Green's research.

On several occasions, both McLean and McIndoe expressed strong concerns to the medical administration about patient safety in relation to Green's experiment. These complaints led to an internal 'whitewash' inquiry.

Green was correct in his assertion that CIS cervix was being overtreated by hysterectomy in the early 1960s, and cone biopsy of the cervix, which had Green's endorsement initially, was a major advance for New Zealand women. However, he progressively became convinced that CIS was not a premalignant condition at all, which led him to oppose cervical cancer screening with the Papanicolaou smear (Pap screening). When evidence from Sweden and Iceland demonstrated decreasing mortality from cervical cancer with regular Pap smear screening, Green's continued failure to acknowledge this fact set the introduction of organised cervical cancer screening in New Zealand back 20 years.

In 1966 Green initiated what can only be described as a controversial experiment. At the time, there was almost universal agreement that CIS was a premalignant lesion. In 1950 the International Federation of Obstetricians and Gynecologists (FIGO), which is responsible for defining the stages of gynaecological cancer, introduced Stage 0 for carcinoma in-situ, implying that it was a premalignant lesion. As a former member of the FIGO Cancer Committee, I am aware that no staging recommendations are made without very strong supporting evidence. In spite of this, Green proposed cytological observation only, for women with biopsy-proven carcinoma *in-situ*. This experiment was accepted by the Hospital Medical Committee, but most women had no idea they were being used as guinea pigs.

Green published a number of reports between 1966 and 1974 to justify his position, but a retrospective review demonstrated that some pathology results had been manipulated to justify his hypothesis. Although Green retired in 1982, his experiment continued, despite the findings of the seminal 1984 paper by McIndoe and his colleagues. This paper clearly demonstrated that women with CIS who continued to have persistent smear abnormalities, irrespective of their initial management, were 25 times more likely to develop invasive cervical cancer than those who had normal follow-up smears.

* * *

It took the attention of feminists and a media response to highlight the tragedy, and the Cartwright Report of 1988 to confirm that an unethical experiment had been carried out on large numbers of women for over 20 years, with disastrous results for many.

It is difficult for an outsider to comprehend how this could have happened. Green was an intelligent but domineering individual, who had no insight into his own limitations. He bullied colleagues who disagreed with him and had the tacit support of his head of department. These circumstances created the 'perfect storm' for a tragedy to happen, and the repercussions are being felt to this day.

When revisionists tried to discredit the Cartwright Report, Professor Ron Jones felt a moral duty to tell the 'inside story' of a saga that had long bedevilled National Women's Hospital. He had endured the silent disapprobation of colleagues who had remained loyal to Green and Bonham, and he kept meticulous records of all written material and conversations relating to the experiment. In addition he became an acknowledged expert in lower genital tract cancers, and was invited to speak on the subject all around the world.

This book is a major contribution to the history of the darkest era in academic medicine in New Zealand. It is written with candour, integrity and wise reflection by an insider who has lived and breathed the controversy for many years. The book provides a portrait of the social environment in which medicine was practised in the second half of the twentieth century;

it acknowledges, also, the state of medical knowledge and the culture of the times; and ultimately comes to the only conclusion possible – Green's 'study' was an unethical experiment on women, which ended for some in cancer and death. Future generations will reflect on this sad era in New Zealand gynaecology with total disbelief.

INTRODUCTION

I swear by Apollo, the healer, Asclepius, Hygieia, and Panacea, and I take witness to all the gods, all the goddesses, to keep according to my ability and judgement, the following Oath and agreement:
To consider dear to me, as my parents, him who taught me this art; to live in common with him and, if necessary, to share my goods with him; to look upon his children as my own brothers, to teach them this art; and that by my teaching, I will impart a knowledge of this art to my own sons, and to my teacher's sons, and to disciples bound by an indenture and oath according to the medical laws, and no others.
I will prescribe regimens for the good of my patients according to my ability and judgement and never do harm to anyone.

HIPPOCRATES OF KOS

THE HIPPOCRATIC OATH PRESENTS doctors with a dilemma – a dilemma that lies at the heart of my story: are doctors responsible first to their teachers and colleagues or to their patients?

When in 1973 I joined the staff of the internationally acclaimed National Women's Hospital (NWH) in Auckland it already had an impressive record in patient care, teaching and research. I was privileged to be working with some of the finest minds in my profession. However, the hospital had a dark secret that was beginning to surface.

Seven years before, in 1966, Associate Professor Herbert Green had begun an experiment that involved following the natural history – that is, not treating – a known cancer precursor, carcinoma *in-situ* (CIS) of the cervix. While the study may have had a laudable aim, Green's views were well out of step with international opinion. Concerns for the outcome for some women in the experiment progressed over time from in-house disagreements to a national scandal. At first I was a silent observer, but eventually I became enmeshed in the resulting controversy.

In my early days at NWH I met Bill McIndoe, an older doctor, who took me into his confidence, sharing his concern about the welfare of an increasing number of women initially presenting with CIS who were later developing invasive cancer. McIndoe plied me with international scientific

13

literature and local documentation relating to cervical cancer. In the end, the hospital's failure to address the concerns relating to Green's experiment led to my co-authoring the 1984 scientific paper that blew the whistle on his work, resulting in public exposure, first by feminist health advocates and then by a judicial inquiry.

The 1987–88 Cervical Cancer Inquiry conducted by Judge (later Dame) Silvia Cartwright, which examined Green's experiment, has had more impact on the practice of medicine in New Zealand than any other single event.[1] In its wake various health-related organisations and universities reflected, reported upon and recommended strategies aimed at preventing similar tragedies. The setting up of a national cervical screening programme, the establishment of a health and disability commissioner and improved ethics committees have been widely welcomed and successful. The incidence of and mortality from cervical cancer have halved since the introduction of the National Cervical Screening Programme in 1990 and results are now comparable with the best in the world.

Although the medical background and chronicle of events leading to the inquiry were well documented by Cartwright, no serious attempt has been made to explore the environment in which Green's research programme took place; the background to what became known as the 'unfortunate experiment'; the relationships between the main characters and the responsibilities of their colleagues. Given the state of medical knowledge of CIS in 1966, how was Green able to convince his colleagues, all of whom treated the precancerous abnormality in accordance with hospital protocols, that he should have their approval to observe the lesion without definitive treatment? Why, when all of the evidence demonstrated he was wrong, did the majority of his colleagues continue to support him? What was the relationship between Green and the senior members of the academic staff at NWH, in particular his head of department, Professor Dennis Bonham? Above all, when evidence of the harm arising from Green's study became known, why did some doctors continue to turn a blind eye and ignore the welfare of his patients?

I recall McIndoe saying during a moment of despair, 'I think Green is mad.' Madness seems to sum up this whole sad affair: that Green gained approval for his study in the first place, against all available evidence; that the study was not halted as the first cancers occurred; that it was not stopped in 1975 at the time an in-house working party examined concerns raised by

McIndoe and Dr Malcolm (Jock) McLean; that Bonham failed to act when he became aware of the outcome of the experiment and, more importantly, following the publication of our damning scientific paper; that Bonham and his loyal supporters and legal advisers did not pause before the inquiry and say, 'Let's look at the evidence – are we defending the indefensible?'; that some members of the medical profession and public continue to this day to demonstrate loyalty to Green; that many members of the medical profession could not say 'I'm sorry'; and that, even today, some individuals continue to rail against the report that resulted from the inquiry.

Recent contentious revisionist viewpoints have caused me to ask myself the same question I asked myself 30 years ago, when I agreed to co-author the scientific paper that exposed Green's experiment: do I not have a responsibility to document truths that will otherwise remain buried in the memories of those of us who worked in the hospital during that time? I knew all of the characters in the story, and I have spent a lifetime continuing to research aspects of the natural history of these cancers. The truth lies in the answer to the question I have repeatedly asked, and revisionists have failed to answer, 'Why did so many women develop cancer?' The answer is simple: Green failed to adequately treat a large group of women with a known precancerous abnormality; many developed cancer and some died.

The significance of Green's experiment has extended well beyond New Zealand. Contrary to Green's personal belief, our studies of his experiment have not only confirmed the significant risk of cancer in women with untreated CIS of the cervix but have, with longer follow-up, provided more precise estimates of the risk.[2] Sadly, Green's experiment is one of the most serious unethical peacetime human experiments of the twentieth century.

Since the Cartwright Inquiry many doctors, nurses, laboratory scientists and patients and families have approached me with their personal stories of the hospital and the experiment. These have been invaluable in forming the framework of this book. Although the events are fresh in the memories of many of us, they occurred in a different age. Similar unrecorded studies no doubt took place in other hospitals and institutions around the world. It was a time when hospitals were ruled by inflexible medical hierarchies; respect for authority, seniority and loyalty were assumed; and bullying and intimidation were commonplace.

It is a story of the frailties of the human condition. Professor Bonham and Associate Professor Green, whose reputations have been so tarnished by the events in this story, both made very significant contributions to the health and welfare of New Zealand women and children. As Shakespeare wrote in *Julius Caesar*, 'The evil that men do lives after them, the good is oft interred with their bones.' The primary responsibility for the outcome of the experiment lies with these two men, but responsibility must be borne by the wider medical fraternity, many of whom were aware of the situation long before we published our 1984 paper. It is also the story of an ill-conceived experiment on a group of unsuspecting women, the lack of empathy for them and their families, and the dichotomy of power and weakness in a group of senior doctors in one of the world's leading obstetric and gynaecological units. It is also the story of a caring profession that has failed to acknowledge the sensitivity, and to some the sacredness, of a woman's genital region. And it is a story of claims and counter-claims, of truths and untruths, and finally, a story of two cancers – one physical, one moral.

My story has evolved from the perspective of a naive young doctor to that of an older, and possibly wiser, man. I did not appreciate what I was letting myself in for when I became involved in a medical dispute involving a group of colleagues from an earlier generation. I have had more than three decades to reflect on my decision to become involved and I know I made the correct decision. However, I still ponder whether the choice of taking the easier path, of turning a blind eye, of remaining silent and loyal to my old colleagues and profession, would have saved me the anguish I experience to this day.

It saddens me to write this book. I am proud of the contributions National Women's Hospital, my hospital, has made to the health and welfare of countless women and children worldwide. There will be those among my colleagues who will view my relating of the home truths as an act of the utmost disloyalty. I need to live with that.

CHAPTER 1

A PROFESSORIAL APPOINTMENT

Vivat academia! Vivant professores!

'Gaudeamus Igitur', traditional
eighteenth-century academic song

I love cricket. Soon after I arrived at National Women's Hospital in the summer of 1973 I was invited to join the cricket team for a local derby match against our neighbour, Greenlane Hospital, whom we played in the adjoining Cornwall Park, under One Tree Hill. The Greenlane players were better attired: most wore whites and cricket boots, and some had colourful old school cricket caps. The NWH side, on the other hand, was less well presented – some players were even in surgical theatre garb – but we had some useful cricketers, including ex-All Black captain Dr Ron Elvidge.

Another notable player was Associate Professor Herbert Green, who for two years had captained his school's 1st XI and, according to local legend, was shod in the battered canvas cricket boots he had worn at school. David Morris – a teammate of mine in the Otago University Cricket XI in the early 1960s, a connoisseur of the game, a batsman of note, a part-time bowler and now a Greenlane Hospital surgeon – was the unfortunate recipient of three straight sixes off his bowling in one over from Green's bat. Wives and girlfriends provided cucumber sandwiches and tea. The afternoon's cricket gave me an early opportunity to meet and socialise with some of my new colleagues.

I felt privileged to have been appointed to a junior specialist position at NWH, an internationally respected unit with a reputation built on the excellence of its current research, clinical teaching and patient care. I had worked in London teaching hospitals made famous for their past achievements but few had earned the current international respect of this youthful New Zealand hospital. I was conscious of being the first 'outside' appointment to the tutor specialist post; previous occupants had spent time in junior training positions in the hospital.

The four senior professors were all well known internationally. Professor Dennis Bonham, the head of the unit, had co-authored the 1958 British Perinatal Mortality Survey, considered by some to be the most important study of its kind in the twentieth century. In 1963 Professor William (Bill) Liley had performed the first successful intrauterine transfusion for rhesus disease, an achievement that hit world headlines in the medical and lay press. Professor Graham (Mont) Liggins, one of only a very small, elite group of New Zealand doctors to be elected as a Fellow of the Royal Society of London, had demonstrated the benefits of antenatal maternal corticosteroids in reducing respiratory distress in premature babies, saving the lives of many thousands of infants worldwide.[1] These projects heralded the beginning of the new field of antenatal therapy. Associate Professor Green had published extensively on his study of untreated carcinoma *in-situ* (CIS) of the cervix, and although there was some uncertainty about the proportion of cases that would progress to cancer, his view was that few or none would do so.[2]

The international status of NWH was in stark contrast to its humble origins in 1946 as the Obstetric and Gynaecological Unit, sited in part of a 1500-bed, single-storey, prefabricated wartime building that had been vacated by the 39th General Hospital of the United States Army. The 123 hospital 'army huts', converted into 48 wards and other facilities, covered a 26-hectare area of Cornwall Park and were linked by a long spinal corridor. While the building was used by the Americans folklore had it that orderlies rode motorbikes in the 800-metre-long corridor; when it was reduced in size, the porters in what became known as Cornwall Hospital cycled between sections. This unit comprised an operating theatre, X-ray facilities and wards with a 135-bed capacity. Another part was converted to a geriatric unit, while much of the original army hospital was either relocated or demolished.

The concept of a national obstetric and gynaecological postgraduate hospital extended back to the 1930s. The New Zealand Obstetric and Gynaecological Society, established in 1927 and spearheaded by the indomitable Dr Doris Gordon, set out to modernise New Zealand obstetric services. In 1929 the society advocated and raised funds for the establishment of a full-time chair in obstetrics and gynaecology at the Otago Medical School and an annual travelling scholarship to enable young New Zealand doctors to specialise in obstetrics and gynaecology overseas.

In 1940 the society agreed that the time had come to set up a postgraduate centre for obstetrics and gynaecology in Auckland to complement the undergraduate centre at Otago University, and that it should be directed 'by a teacher of empire standing'.[3] This idea led to considerable friction between the Otago and Auckland University authorities.

In 1943 the Auckland mayor, Sir Ernest Davis, headed a large deputation to inform Minister of Health Arnold Nordmeyer that 'an influential body of citizens will undertake to raise a substantial sum to ensure the creation of a centre in Auckland for the postgraduate study of obstetrics and gynaecology'.[4] By 1947 a public appeal, led by the Rotary Club, and with Doris Gordon again providing the impetus, had raised the enormous sum of £101,231 to endow a chair, and the first professor, South African Gerald Spence-Smythe, was appointed in 1952. He resigned three years later and returned to Johannesburg, complaining that 'there was no department, no lecture room, no laboratory, no assistant, nothing of my own'.[5] The renamed National Women's Hospital appointed Harvey Carey as its second professor. He is credited with establishing its reputation, particularly recognising the potential talents of young researchers such as Liley and Liggins. However, Carey's dual role as professor and medical director created insurmountable difficulties that eventually led to a division of control between an Auckland Hospital Board-appointed medical superintendent and a university-appointed professor. In addition there were the almost inevitable conflicts between some clinicians of the existing establishment ('town') and the new university order ('gown'). These were the principal catalysts leading to Carey's resignation and subsequent appointment to the Chair of Obstetrics and Gynaecology at the Royal Women's Hospital, Sydney.

Late in 1962 advertisements for the postgraduate chair vacated by Carey were placed in medical journals and newspapers throughout Britain, Australia, South Africa, the United States and New Zealand.[6] Dr Harold Francis, a young New Zealand academic in Liverpool, applied but later withdrew; and Dr Douglas Robb, the Chancellor of Auckland University, asked Dr Bernard Kyle, who had been assistant medical director under Carey, to apply. He, however, declined the invitation, having already committed himself to a part-time visiting position on the NWH staff, and to private practice.[7] Finally two applicants were considered: Dr Dennis Bonham from England and Dr Herbert Green from Auckland.

Dr Dennis Geoffrey Bonham possessed impressive credentials. Following education at King Edward VI Grammar School, Nuneaton, he went up to Cambridge University for his undergraduate degree and completed his medical training at University College Hospital, London, in 1948. He spent the next 14 years in London and southern England doing postgraduate training in surgery, obstetrics and gynaecology. This time included three years of national service at Fighter Command Headquarters, Bentley Priory. He became a Member of the Royal College of Obstetricians and Gynaecologists (MRCOG) in 1955, and in 1958 a Fellow of the Royal College of Surgeons of England (FRCS). He returned to University College Hospital as a first assistant and not only extended his clinical experience but also became immersed in the academic milieu. He had succeeded in becoming a product of the fiercely competitive, paternalistic, hierarchical British medical system and was now ready for a senior academic or consultant post.

Professor Will Nixon, one of Britain's leading obstetricians in the 1950s and 1960s, recognised Bonham's research potential and chose him to partner Dr Neville Butler in taking responsibility for the organisation of the 1958 British Perinatal Mortality Survey. Butler and Bonham designed, planned, analysed and reported on a study of virtually every birth in England, Scotland and Wales occurring over one week, and the neonatal deaths within the same group for the next three months.[8] Ethics committees did not exist at the time, and neither did the concept of informed consent, but medical confidentiality was considered important and extended to the use of medical information for this type of research.

In the precomputer era, Butler, Bonham, his wife Nancie and his father laboured on the data long into the nights and at weekends. Those who later knew Bonham's capacity for work would understand his comment that Butler would come to his home in the evening after a day of clinical duties and they would toil through until breakfast. Thus 17,205 births and 666 deaths were studied. In a prepublication press conference late in 1962 Nixon appealed for improved care for mothers and babies. His emotional comments hit the headlines: 'If we had 50 deaths a week from air crashes something would be done, yet there are 50 babies a week dying of preventable asphyxia.'[9] The British Perinatal Report, finally published in 1963, was Bonham's crowning achievement. This research alone would have swayed an appointment committee anxious to improve the standard of maternity services in New Zealand.

Ironically it was Bonham, not Green, who first became involved in investigating normal and abnormal changes in the cervix. In 1961 Bonham participated in a symposium at the Royal Society of Medicine in London, presenting a paper on his research on the physiological and pathological changes to the pregnant and postnatal cervix. Bonham commented on the natural history (the outcome in the absence of treatment) of cervical 'erosion' and discussed the early diagnosis of CIS of the cervix. He observed that obstetricians and gynaecologists 'have both a great responsibility and a unique opportunity of screening our patients [with smear tests]', and lamented the poor cytology facilities in Britain.[10] The discussion of his paper was led by Professor Hugh McLaren from Birmingham, who would later vigorously debate the natural history of CIS of the cervix with Herbert Green.

Bonham also became involved in basic laboratory studies involving examination of vaginal fluid for enzymes thought to be associated with cervical cancer and precancer, which was seen as a possible alternative screening test to the Pap smear (see p. 00).[11] He was supported in his research by the British Empire Cancer Campaign. He pursued these studies after coming to New Zealand, but the test was ultimately discarded because it was non-specific.[12] In applying for the position at NWH, 39-year-old Bonham was following the advice of his mentor, Professor Nixon, who recommended to aspiring young academics they should follow his example and, at least initially, 'Go east, young man.'[13] Soon after his arrival in New Zealand, Bonham contributed an article for the *Family Planning Association Journal* in which he observed: 'Death from carcinoma of the cervix could be eliminated in this country before the end of the century.'[14] This was one of 12 similar quotes from articles written in the 1960s which Green distributed to students to emphasise the prevailing international opinions regarding the benefits of cervical screening.[15]

The second candidate for the chair, Dr George Herbert Green, came from a South Otago farming background and received his secondary education at South Otago High School in Balclutha, where he was head boy. In 1935 he entered Dunedin Teachers' College and studied part time at Otago University, completing a BA in 1938 and a BSc in 1940. He also worked part time in Sir Horace Smirk's laboratory at the medical school. This broad education prepared him for medicine, teaching, research and his later interest in medical history. Green entered Otago Medical School in

1941 and graduated in 1945. Companions at Knox College remember him as being older, rather grumpy and a heavy cigarillo smoker.[16] He used his height and well-built frame to advantage, particularly in rugby and cricket. His teammates in the University Senior B rugby team frequently needed to restrain him when he repeatedly disputed refereeing decisions.[17] Green's combative nature was already established.

After spending two years as a house surgeon in Dunedin, Green moved to Auckland to begin his specialist training in obstetrics and gynaecology at Cornwall (later National Women's) Hospital. It was during this time he first became interested in the study of cervical cancer and its pathology; in 1949 he wrote his MRCOG commentary on 'The early diagnosis of cervical cancer'. He also remembered being influenced by the distress of one of his Balclutha school teachers who had developed cervical cancer.[18]

The old Cornwall Hospital building was a haven for fertile stray cats. Professor Barbara Heslop, then a sixth-year medical student, recalled Green spaying stray female cats on the operating theatre table during the evenings – 'cat gynaecology'. Nursing staff prepared a 'cat instrument tray', medical students caught three or four cats per session, gave the anaesthetic and were instructed to spray escaping fleas with ethyl chloride and remove them with forceps from the operating table. The theatre was then cleaned in preparation for the following day's human surgery. This, Heslop noted, was 'Herb's idea of a social service and I guess we concurred. If this sort of thing happened today, questions would be asked in parliament! In so many respects it was truly another age.'[19] Dr Algar Warren, Green's fellow resident at Cornwall and later medical superintendent of NWH, told the story of a nurse who was persuaded to have an X-ray with a pillowcase filled with kittens lying on her abdomen for a joke. Dr Tony Crick, the radiologist called to interpret the X-ray, was understandably initially perplexed by the appearance but, on seeing minute bones arrayed as several tiny tails, he recognised he had been duped.[20]

Green left the Obstetric and Gynaecological Unit at the end of 1950 and worked briefly in private practice in order to raise money for travel to Britain to further his postgraduate experience. He passed his MRCOG in 1951 but later failed the primary FRCS examination.[21] After almost a year of locum practice he was appointed to a two-year position as a senior registrar at the West Middlesex Hospital. New Zealander Dr Bob Gudex, who was a fellow resident, noted that Green was a good leader and teacher, and an innovator – for example, he introduced routine weighing of antenatal patients. Gudex also noted Green 'was never afraid to voice his opinion'.[22] This characteristic was illustrated some years later when a colleague, Dr Ian Barrowclough, was demonstrating how to apply a pair of obstetric forceps. Overhearing the description, Green rushed forward, grabbed the forceps out of Barrowclough's hands and without so much as an 'Excuse me', said, 'This is the way you do it!'[23] Before returning to New Zealand Green spent seven months in Dr Stanley Way's gynaecological cancer unit in Newcastle, where, in addition to his clinical work, he undertook study in cytology.

There were no academic positions available in New Zealand when Green returned, so he accepted the first specialist obstetric and gynaecological position at Wanganui Hospital. General practitioners and house surgeons there remembered him with fondness and as an enthusiastic teacher who was keen to improve local obstetric services.[24] Green quite correctly felt he had a responsibility to audit these services, although his review of the indications for caesarean section was not received kindly by the hospital's general surgeons, who shared this surgery with him.[25] In 1956, encouraged by Carey, Green returned to NWH, and this enabled him to pursue his interest in cervical cancer. In his words, his early experiences with the disease caused him 'to want to seek a means by which this particular type of cancer could be prevented'.[26]

* * *

In 1963 Bonham and Green were interviewed by two separate committees for the postgraduate chair in obstetrics and gynaecology – Bonham in London, Green in Auckland.

In London Dr John Foster, secretary of the Association of Universities of the British Commonwealth (AUBC), convened a committee to interview Bonham. It comprised Sir John Peel, Surgeon-Gynaecologist to Queen Elizabeth II, as chairman, Dr John Stallworthy, a New Zealander and senior obstetrician and gynaecologist in Oxford, and Foster himself.[27] Coincidentally, the Auckland University chancellor, Dr Douglas Robb, Auckland's most powerful medical man, and vice-chancellor, Kenneth Maidment, were in London attending an AUBC meeting; they interviewed Bonham separately from the committee.

Together with Doris Gordon, Douglas Robb was one of the driving forces behind the establishment and endowment of NWH. There is a striking parallel between Robb's early experience as a surgeon, his description of 'naked personal power politics', and the events about to unfold in this book. Keen to improve surgical standards, Robb performed audits of surgical outcomes on several organs, including the uterus.[28] His audit of rectal cancer pointed to serious shortcomings by some senior surgeons and, 'in the climate of presumed surgical infallibility then common, this was much resented'.[29] On the advice of these senior colleagues, the Hospital Board declined to reappoint Robb to his surgical position at Auckland Hospital at the time of his review in 1935. His friend, poet A.R.D. Fairburn, wrote a poem dedicated to him entitled 'To a Friend in the Wilderness'. Robb remained in the wilderness until 1942 when the board acknowledged his sterling qualities and he was reappointed. As his obituarist, Dr David Cole, observed, '[h]istorians will probably see the assertion by an idealistic surgeon of the need for scientific accountability and the consequential harsh retaliatory reassertion of power by the establishment, as a point of some significance in medical practice in this country'.[30]

Green was interviewed by Robb and Maidment before they went to London and then by the Auckland Obstetric and Gynaecological Academic Advisory Committee. This comprised pro-chancellor Henry Cooper (chair), the acting vice-chancellor (not named), Dr Michael Gilmour, obstetricians Dr Geoffrey Fisher, Dr Jefcoate Harbutt and Dr Bruce Grieve, and superintendent-in-chief Dr Wilton Henley.[31] Dr Arthur Bell, past president of the Royal College of Obstetricians and Gynaecologists, happened to be in Auckland and was invited to join the discussion.

At the time of his interview, Green had been first assistant to Professor Carey for seven years and had been elevated to associate professorial status in 1962. The reason for his promotion to a level that traditionally reflects academic achievement is unclear, since he lacked a significant academic background and had few research publications. He had, however, been awarded a Lederle International Fellowship for 1962, which allowed him to study for eight months in the Department of Obstetrics and Gynecology at Columbia University, New York. His immediate aim was 'to find out something about the distribution of preinvasive cervical cancer in the intact uterus' (that is, a cervix not disturbed by diagnostic biopsy). He later wrote, 'I brought [the uteruses] with me and never once did I think of what I would say if a customs officer asked me to open the container and explain the contents!'[32] Later, lawyers at the Cartwright Inquiry would refer to these as 'flying uteruses'. It is not known exactly how Green obtained these uteruses; in those days pathology specimens were regarded as the property of the laboratory. Cervical cancer was found in the uterus of one unfortunate woman and Green wrote back to inform NWH staff of the diagnosis; the 32-year-old woman died soon after.

Green had proven himself to be a good teacher and was popular with colleagues, who frequently entrusted him with the care of their wives. He enjoyed battling for the underdog, and patients or colleagues who needed special assistance could count on his personal support. He lobbied successfully for the continued independence and identity of the postgraduate school when the Auckland Medical School opened in 1968.

Until the 1970s a fellowship of a Royal College of Surgeons, in addition to a membership of a Royal College of Obstetricians and Gynaecologists, was considered a significant advantage for those seeking senior positions in teaching hospitals: Green's lack of an FRCS would have counted against him. In the past some professorial candidates in New Zealand had been invited to demonstrate their surgical skills to members of the visiting staff and in this situation some more academically talented individuals elected to withdraw their candidature. It remains unknown how much the appointment committees considered factors such as the interpersonal skills and personalities of the applicants. Green was liked and supported by the obstetricians on the Auckland interviewing committee. Bonham, having ruffled a few feathers among his London colleagues, was not as well respected.[33] Although Green had local support – 'honest Herb … a Kiwi doing research'[34] – the Auckland committee went along with the opinion of the London group, and Maidment and Robb. Their decision was cabled to Auckland:

Chancellor has interviewed Bonham fully.

Joint recommendation of Chancellor and Vice-Chancellor agrees with AUBC and Vice-Chancellor's personal letter that Bonham is outstanding and should be appointed at once. Monash [University] appointment imminent and likely to favour Bonham.[35]

Despite missing out on the chair, Green retained academic respect and was appointed to the Medical Research Council. In 1968–69 he chaired the committee examining 'The adequacy of medical statistics in New Zealand'.[36] There was an irony here, as Green had stated that he was not a statistician – it was Bonham who lectured on the topic, having gained extensive experience while working on the British Perinatal Mortality Survey.

***

I first met Herb Green in 1973, a decade after he had been passed over for the chair. He was obviously still bitter and told me that while local specialists had supported him, Robb had 'knifed me in the back': he had learned of Bonham's appointment in a newspaper. By this time he had been an associate professor for 11 years, was settled in Auckland and had not applied for professorial posts elsewhere. One can only assume Green recognised he had to co-exist with Bonham as his new head of department. Their uneasy relationship was obvious not only to those of us working in the hospital but also to outsiders.[37] I suspect they had a tacit understanding not to interfere in each other's fields of interest. Bonham soon ceased his cervical cancer research, leaving this to Green, and focused on other research, university administration, and clinical and teaching commitments. He continued to work on the safety of obstetric care and was always willing to encourage and support others in their research.

Green was a tall, balding man with a shambling gait. It appeared incongruous when, having been driven to work by his petite wife, Joan, he would unfold his large frame from the passenger seat of his Mini Cooper car. Medical men in the 1950s and 1960s were generally socially conservative, many becoming more liberal as society changed from the 1970s, but Green remained conservative to the end of his career. Although he had no known religious affiliation, he supported neither sterilisation nor abortion. His conservative approach to the former was illustrated in a paper he wrote on tubal ligation early in his career, in which he emphasised the risks but made no acknowledgement of the benefits.[38] Later he did admit, however, to having sterilised women where he believed it was justified.[39] On the topic of termination of pregnancy the four academic seniors in the postgraduate department were divided in their views: Bonham and Liggins were liberal, Liley and Green conservative – in fact Liley was president of the Society for the Protection of the Unborn Child (SPUC). Green took a dim view of societal liberalisation and the establishment of a private abortion clinic in Auckland in 1974. The following year he set out his views to Dr John Dobson, a representative of the Australia and New Zealand College of Psychiatrists:

Perhaps I oversimplify the matter of abortion but, to me, the question of abortion of a normal pregnancy is a moral one and has nothing to do with the practice of medicine. My thoughts on the matter are governed entirely by the fact that I cannot possibly see how the social and economic circumstances of one human being can be of more importance than the life of another. Therefore, all such arguments I have adduced in the way of complications of abortion are strictly irrelevant to the main issue.[40]

The Contraception, Sterilisation and Abortion Act 1977 permitted abortions to be performed in public hospitals or in private hospitals licensed under the Hospitals Act 1957. Women with complications following termination of pregnancy at a private abortion clinic were referred to NWH for further management. Although every attempt was made to ensure such cases were placed under a team of liberal gynaecologists, these women were sometimes admitted under less liberal on-call consultants who were, understandably, unhappy to receive them. On one occasion Green made a statutory declaration with the police regarding a patient with post-termination complications who was admitted under his care. On the basis of the complaint the police prosecutor had no choice but to advise the police to obtain a search warrant for the private abortion clinic in order to investigate the matter. This led to the high-profile trial and eventual acquittal of the principal operating doctor, James Woolnough.[41] Green also discussed with the medical school dean, Professor David Cole, the standing of John Werry, the professor of psychiatry: Green felt Werry should not be performing abortions, presumably because he was not a gynaecologist.[42]

A generation of nurses remembers Green for his obstetric teaching. His book *Introduction to Obstetrics* went through four editions between 1962 and 1982. He used the English royalties to buy, unseen, a late-1920s Rolls Royce, which he had shipped back to New Zealand.[43]

Green was trained in the old school of operative obstetrics in the 1940s and 1950s, where he had learned difficult manipulative and forceps deliveries, something he enjoyed demonstrating to students and house surgeons. As a house surgeon, Professor Rod Jackson recalls being told to go to the delivery theatre and 'see something you will never see again – Professor Green is about to perform the vaginal delivery of breech triplets!'[44] By the 1970s progress demanded more caesarean sections, not only for the sake of the mother but also for the fetus. When I was tutor specialist, from 1973 to 1975, I was chastised by Green for resorting to caesarean section earlier than he considered necessary. His large hands and fingers were not ideally suited to such surgical procedures.

Green held some unconventional views and unrealistic expectations. Later in his career he became absorbed by royal obstetric tragedies and published a number of papers on the subject.[45] He believed that Jane Seymour, third wife of Henry VIII, had been delivered of an infant by caesarean section. Extraordinarily, and unsuccessfully, he sought permission from the Queen and the RCOG to exhume her embalmed body in order to look for evidence of a scar.[46] In reviewing Green's paper 'A royal obstetric tragedy', Professor Sir John Dewhurst, a former president of the RCOG in London, noted a number of errors that he considered affected the quality of scholarship. He described Green as a 'selective historian' who left out evidence that did not suit his argument.[47]

Vivian Bartley Green-Armytage, a noted London obstetrician and gynaecologist, presented a rare, 1754 first edition of William Smellie's *Anatomical Tables* to the Postgraduate School of Obstetrics and Gynaecology on the occasion of its founding in 1951. Green had a beautiful facsimile produced, the proceeds from the sale going to the department research fund.

Green and Bonham were fiercely loyal to NWH and, in particular, to the Postgraduate School of Obstetrics and Gynaecology. When there was a choice between 'town and gown', they made no secret of their support for the latter. When the Mater Misericordiae Hospital maternity unit closed in 1979 there was widespread dismay from the public and medical profession. The *Auckland Star* published an article describing the Mater as 'a place where people were referred to by their name'.[48] This drew a swift response from Green, who said there was no case for seeing the Mater as having provided a higher level of care than NWH. In 1969 he had written to a patient who had shifted to Wellington stating, 'unfortunately [there is] no equivalent to National Women's Hospital in Wellington!'[49]

Bonham was a large, bald-headed man – once described as a 'colossus'[50] – with boundless energy and vision, who lived and breathed hospital. He took his teaching responsibilities seriously, never comprehending why junior medical staff did not wish to attend weekend ward rounds when they were not on duty. He was a complex individual with an overbearing and difficult personality. In Bonham's obituary, Professor John Scott observed that 'he strode through the effect of much opposition from people he perceived to be less able than himself and earned a reputation for arrogance.[51] In part this may have reflected shortcomings in his social skills, which had been recognised long before he left London.

Like Bonham, Dr Don Menzies and Dr Denis Hawkins (later Professor of Obstetrics and Gynaecology at the University of London) were full-time assistants to Professor Nixon at University College Hospital from 1962 to 1964: both described Bonham as bombastic and a bully. Menzies pointed out that Bonham 'did not quite fit in' and was 'perhaps uneasy with his background', and that 'midwives disliked his style of man management'.[52] Scott noted that Bonham 'was not afraid of academic controversy: he was usually well prepared to meet arguments of the opposition, with bluntness rather than tact characterising his professional style'.[53] Professor John Werry recalled a meeting with representatives from the Family Planning Association and senior teachers, instigated by Bonham, to discuss the controversial aspects of sex education in schools contained in the 1977 Johnson Report. Bonham was so incensed by one teacher's lack of understanding of the content that he stood up, threw the report at the poor man and said, 'Read it!'[54]

* * *

I first encountered Bonham early in January 1973, the beginning of my three-year term as a junior specialist at NWH. I was passing behind some queues of women waiting in the outpatients department to arrange their next appointment when I heard a loud voice approaching from an adjacent corridor. The owner of the voice was a large man in a fresh white coat, wisps of dark, Brylcreemed hair combed over his bald pate. He was obviously very agitated. Not only was he shouting, but he was also progressively dismembering a set of patient records, sending sheets of paper flying in his wake. His outrage was the result of incorrect filing of a patient's records. He was in full flight to remonstrate with Miss Dynes, the senior medical records officer. Neither I nor I suspect the open-mouthed crowd of women had ever witnessed a doctor act in this manner. Clearly this was not an opportune time to introduce myself. I slunk away to the non-professorial clinic awaiting a more propitious time to make the professor's acquaintance.

Others encountered Bonham's tantrums and predilection for dismembering patient files. As a trainee intern Dr Jeanie McDonald was 'incredibly intimidated' by him. On one occasion she witnessed an altercation between Bonham and an unfortunate woman house surgeon. 'Bonham snatched the patient notes and threw them out an upper-storey window. I watched as the unbound pages came apart and fluttered to the ground below.'[55]

His professorial position and difficult character isolated him from many colleagues. Junior medical staff were often terrified of him, although in my experience he generally backed down when someone stood up to him. Dr Jock Carnachan recalled Bonham once becoming increasingly angry at the shortcomings in the collective knowledge of a group of house surgeons. 'He flew into a rage, threw his notes on the desk and kicked the chair in front of him. This was immediately followed by a howl of pain and he limped out and left us to it.'[56] When Dr Chris Hoskins, a consultant in Edmonton, Canada, declined a registrar position offered him by Bonham, the latter said he would make sure Hoskins got no further position in New Zealand.[57]

Some stood up to Bonham. One who did was infamous NWH 'house surgeon' Milan Brych, a Czechoslovakian refugee who claimed to have been a medically qualified 'chest physician' in his own country (see Chapter 5). Jock Carnachan was in the staff tearoom when Bonham swept in with his entourage and expressed his surprise at seeing a former 'chest physician', smoking a cigarette; he advised him to stop. Brych responded immediately: 'So you are giving up sex, Professor Bonham? You see, smoking is also one of my pleasures.' In Carnachan's words, 'The assembled gathering awaited Bonham's response, but he was speechless and the expectation gave way to general mirth.'[58]

In 1980 my wife, Barbara, and I attended an RCOG congress soirée at the Royal Scottish Academy in Edinburgh. A man who had seen 'Auckland' on my name badge introduced himself and asked if I knew Professor Bonham, whom he had not seen since sharing a school dormitory with him as a young teenager. When he described what he thought Bonham might be like more than 40 years later, his description matched perfectly the man I knew.[59]

Bonham had a genuine wish to improve the health of New Zealand women. His background in national perinatal research served him well in this desire, as New Zealand's obstetric and perinatal services needed significant improvement. His style of leadership was not universally admired, but he got things done. He travelled the length and breadth of New Zealand observing how maternity services were being run and advising the Health

Department on initiatives to improve maternal and infant care. Many small maternity units were closed, often with considerable local opposition, maternal mortality declined and perinatal mortality fell from 22.3 per 1000 in 1965 to 16.5 per 1000 in 1975, and to 7.5 per 1000 in 1990.[60] Perinatal epidemiology remained the focal point of Bonham's academic interest: he founded the New Zealand Perinatal Society in 1980 and was an adviser to the World Health Organization Maternal and Child Health Committee.

Throughout his time at NWH Bonham chaired the monthly perinatal mortality meetings. Staff attendance was compulsory, even though meetings were held on Saturday mornings or Monday evenings. Every case was discussed in detail and individual staff were left in no doubt when shortcomings were identified in their care of individual patients. With Bonham's support, Green supported many Asian and Pacific Island doctors coming to NWH for postgraduate studies, introducing them to European-style medicine and a New Zealand way of life. Professor Jong Duk Kim from South Korea recalled his time at the hospital with 'mixed fear, respect and gratitude'.[61] He was instructed to report his weekend activities to Bonham on a Monday.

Although they had their differences, Bonham and Green also had much in common. Both were large-framed men whom many found both physically and intellectually intimidating. A secretary in the medical library had vivid memories of her telephone conversations with them. 'In the mid-1970s we were totally reliant on the post for letters, journals and books. Most library users were polite and understanding when a journal or book was delayed in the post. There were however two exceptions – Professors Bonham and Green – and both have left a lasting impression on me; they were demanding, impatient, arrogant and rude.'[62]

Both men were bullies and Green could be extremely stubborn. Michael Churchouse, charge cytotechnologist at NWH, described Green as 'a big man with a deep, loud, gruff voice, and somewhat invincible – quite a bully in fact, and peers and lesser mortals did not cross swords with him lightly'.[63] Professor Rod Jackson, who observed Bonham and Green during his time as a medical student and house surgeon, found them to be 'insensitive, arrogant, patronising, unpleasant people'.[64] Both men were products of the patriarchal, authoritarian medical system of the time, and both were academically ambitious. Professor Innes Asher was attached to the Bonham–Green team as a medical student in 1971. She 'felt distinctly uncomfortable in [Bonham's] presence'. To the 'chosen few he was incredibly nice, but to most of the students his body language, inappropriate and unprofessional behaviour made me sense he abused his power and position'. By contrast she warmed to Green, who demonstrated 'universal kindness to his patients, staff and students'.[65]

I believe Green enjoyed being a devil's advocate and sceptic – he called himself a 'doubting Thomas'.[66] The *Auckland Star* described him as being 'sceptical about links between the anti-miscarriage drug DES [diethylstilboestrol] and vaginal cancers in the daughters of women who used it' – even though the links were well established by that time.[67] Professor Richard Doll, in his concluding remarks at an Auckland epidemiology symposium in 1973, acknowledged Green's reference, in his own paper, to 'stirring the pot'.[68] Dr Liam Wright, the surgeon who worked with Green for many years, described him as a bully, 'a man with inflexible views who enjoyed being different … a man who would never admit he was wrong', and observed that if one's views differed from Green's 'the discussion inevitably became unpleasant'.[69] 'Don't confuse me with the facts, my mind is already made up', a quotation reputedly written on Green's office blackboard by Dr Bevan Reid of Sydney, was there for as long as I can remember. Mont Liggins recorded this in an article marking Green's retirement from the university and many staff members recalled it.[70]

While Green displayed the male chauvinism typical of his generation, Bonham held liberal views on the place of women in society: he was an enthusiastic supporter of women in medicine. At a heads of department meeting at the Auckland Medical School in the mid-1970s some professors suggested that, because of the ever-increasing numbers and proportion of women medical graduates, the numbers of female entrants should be restricted. The discussion was quickly quashed when Bonham stood up and, in typically forthright fashion, championed the cause and the rights of women medical students and graduates.[71]

An insight into the relationship between Green and Bonham emerges from the following observation of a general practitioner/obstetrician, Dr Henry Doerr. He was among a group of GPs with a Diploma of Obstetrics who, from the mid-1970s to the late 1980s, delivered 70–80 babies a year, most of them at NWH, and hence had 'a reasonable amount of contact with both Professors Green and Bonham'. He never forgot one particular confinement:

I delivered one of my patients, a first-time mother, and she and her husband were ecstatic with their new baby boy. Unfortunately the joy quickly turned to anguish, when, shortly after the birth, it became apparent the child had Down's syndrome. Over the next day or two [we' discovered] the child also had duodenal atresia, a condition requiring corrective surgery in the next few days or it would prove fatal. These first-time parents faced an agonising dilemma – to permit surgery and raise a child with Down's syndrome, or to refuse surgery and allow their child to die.

After 'several intense discussions' and 'agonising over the ethics of the case and reflecting on their own religious and moral values', the 'intelligent and articulate couple' decided against surgery.

During this stressful decision-making process several National Women's Hospital staff members, none of whom had any clinical responsibility for the woman's care, kept coming uninvited to her single room with the clear intention of trying to get her to agree to surgery. Naturally these visits – frequent, unsolicited and unwelcome – added to the stress of this new mother. I learned that these visits were orchestrated by Professor Green. Although he never visited my patient or discussed her care with me, he organised his 'cadre' of staff to try to influence the couple's decision.

As a GP obstetrician, I felt I was no match for Professor Green: instead I alerted Professor Bonham to my patient's difficulties, fully explaining the circumstances and the unwelcome intrusions. He told me he would take care of it. I do not know what took place subsequent to our discussion, but I do know the interference stopped immediately.[72]

Green's dress, deportment, social skills and outside interests identified him with his farming roots: he enjoyed restoring vintage cars. Bonham's life was dominated by the hospital, although later he became interested in growing orchids. Patients often warmed to Green's reassuring, fatherly manner. Sister Isobel Fisher, who cared for Green's cancer patients in Ward 9, adored him and treasured a cup and saucer he gave her when she retired.[73]

Liggins, Liley and Green were not only senior academic departmental colleagues who occasionally collaborated on scientific papers; they were also friends who jointly owned, with John Groome, a 200-hectare forestry venture north of Auckland. This required not only mutual investment and understanding but also considerable energy.

* * *

Unsurprisingly Green, eight years Bonham's senior and the local candidate who had failed to be appointed to the chair, did not embrace his rival's arrival in Auckland. And Bonham made matters worse for himself when, in the English custom, he began his first letter to his soon-to-be assistant with the words 'Dear Green'.[74] The pair probably first met in Brisbane where Bonham, en route to New Zealand, gave a paper at a conference that Green also attended. When Bonham arrived in Auckland in December 1963, he had achieved his life's ambition to become professor and head of department of a unit with considerable potential. He was conscious he had to build on the foundation established by his predecessor, Harvey Carey, and would have been aware of the considerable challenge of restructuring New Zealand's maternity services. He was, however, unaware of his greatest challenge – establishing a professional relationship with Green, the man whom he had defeated in his quest for the chair, the man who would ultimately destroy his career.

CHAPTER 2

THE EVOLUTION OF A MISBELIEF ...

The evidence seems almost certain that preinvasive cancer if left untreated will progress to invasive cancer. Exceptionally, some cases may regress.

HERBERT GREEN, 1957

Carcinoma in-situ *is probably benign in the great majority of cases.*

HERBERT GREEN, 1964

The patient with in-situ *cancer has only the normal chance of developing future invasive cancer.*

HERBERT GREEN, 1970

ADVANCES IN MEDICINE often follow a common pattern: a chance observation leading to independent confirmation and finally, after a lengthy period of scientific evaluation, acceptance and introduction into everyday practice. Throughout the process there are sceptics who challenge new theories and practices and, in so doing, play an important role in focusing attention on potential shortcomings in the 'new truth'. The almost universal acceptance of the precancerous potential of CIS of the cervix followed this path.

The idea that cervical cancer developed in 'precancerous' tissue was first reported in the prestigious 1886 Harveian Lecture by Dr John Williams, physician accoucheur to Queen Victoria's family, who delivered the future Edward VIII and George VI. He was also an obstetrician at Bonham's alma mater, University College Hospital, London. Williams reported the chance microscopic finding in an asymptomatic woman, noting that the abnormality 'may remain superficial for a long time'.[1]

A decade later, a number of European authors began reporting their clinical and microscopic observations of women with white patches (leukoplakia) on the cervix, some of which progressed to cancer.[2] In 1908 W. Schauenstein in Germany was the first to report a detailed assessment of the pathology of the cervix, proposing that invasive cervical cancer developed in 'atypical' epithelium (superficial cell layer). Two years later Isidore Rubin, in New York, described 'incipient carcinoma' and considered the differences between the normal cervix, atypical epithelium that might eventually progress to cancer, and cancer.[3] In questioning how pathologists could define the differences between benign, precancerous and malignant cervical tissue, Rubin suggested that once these differences were clearly defined it might be possible to prevent cervical cancer: this was the first time the possibility of cervical cancer prevention had been raised. Although pathologists increasingly recognised the similarities in the appearance and arrangement of cells in the preinvasive and invasive stages of cervical cancer, some did not recognise the preinvasive phase as a separate biological entity until the 1930s.

The introduction of universally acceptable pathology definitions and terminology for atypical cervical epithelium were catalysts for progress. In 1932 A.C. Broders introduced the term 'carcinoma in-situ' to describe the presence of malignant cells through the entire thickness of the epithelial surface without invasion below the basement membrane.[4] The varied descriptive terminology for lesions less abnormal than CIS created confusion and in the early 1950s J.W. Reagan and his colleagues introduced the term 'dysplasia' to designate those abnormalities with pathological features that were intermediate between normal epithelium and early invasive cancer.[5] Ralph Richart's introduction of the cervical intraepithelial neoplasia (CIN) 1, 2, 3 terminology in 1966 both unified the existing dysplasia/CIS terminology and introduced the concept of a pathological and biological continuum.[6] Today CIS is included, with severe dysplasia, in cervical intraepithelial neoplasia 3 (CIN 3) terminology.

The most compelling circumstantial evidence of the precancerous origin of cervical cancer noted by early investigators was the similarity between the appearance and arrangement of microscopic cells in precancer and invasive cancer compared with normal epithelial tissue. Early invasive cancers always arose in CIS, and more advanced cancers often had CIS at the margin.[7] Green stressed this point in his early lecture notes but failed to mention it in his publications, presumably because as time went on it did not fit easily with his changing beliefs.[8] In addition to epidemiological evidence, new and exciting laboratory evidence – from histochemistry, electron-microscopy, cytogenetics and molecular biology – has continued to support the concept that cervical cancer arises in a precursor lesion – CIS.

For the two decades from the mid-1930s, and before the introduction of the cervical smear – Pap test – increasing numbers of clinical reports supported the conclusions of the earlier microscopic observations. In the United States in 1934, four women with invasive cervical cancer, on review, were noted to have had CIS in biopsies performed three to 12 years earlier;[9] a prospective experiment on women with untreated CIS was terminated in 1938 after numbers of these precursor lesions were observed to progress to cervical cancer.[10] In Norway, 34 (26 per cent) of 127 women with untreated cervical 'precancerosis' (CIS) who had been diagnosed in the years 1930–50 developed cancer during a 15-year follow-up.[11]

Dr George Papanicolaou, a Greek émigré to the United States, is usually credited with the origin of the cervical smear (Pap) test.[12] This simple cytology test involves scraping cells from the surface of the cervix or vagina, staining them and examining them under a microscope to search for abnormalities. The first description of vaginal smears, however, was by a Romanian, Aureli Babes, in 1927.[13] Papanicolaou's early research involved monitoring the changes in appearance of vaginal cells during the hormonal fluctuations of the menstrual cycle – the source of the daily samples for his research was his long-suffering wife. He changed the direction of his cytological research from hormonal changes to potential cancer detection when he was advised this would attract better funding. Papanicolaou was nominated on five occasions for a Nobel Prize but was always unsuccessful; it is not certain whether he was familiar with Babes' earlier publication.[14] The Nobel committee possibly took the view that Papanicolaou may have been aware of Babes' description but failed to acknowledge it.[15]

The introduction of the Pap smear test in the 1950–60s brought dramatic change. It was now possible to detect and treat precancerous cervical cells in healthy, asymptomatic women with clinically normal cervices. Boyes, Fidler and Lock, three Canadian researchers, reasoned that Pap screening a population of women, and treating and removing abnormalities such as CIS, should lead to a reduction in the incidence of cervical cancer. Over 12 years they screened and treated abnormalities in approximately one-third of British Columbian women over the age of 20, and between 1955 and 1960 the incidence of cervical cancer decreased by 30 per cent.[16] Green vigorously challenged this and other screening studies, citing the falling incidence of cervical cancer before the introduction of screening. This phenomenon did confuse the picture and make evaluation of screening more difficult. The fall appears to have been partly the result of changing sexual mores.[17]

Green was not alone in being cautious about endorsing population screening. A number of epidemiologists, including high-profile British academics Richard Doll, Archie Cochrane and George Knox, were aware of the previously uncounted harms of screening and the need for evidence to demonstrate its effectiveness.[18] Knox, writing in 1966, the year Green began his experiment, observed that 'the fact that ... [cytology] has not yet won the determined support necessary for an effective preventative measure is not due entirely to ignorance, apathy and expense'. There was, he wrote, 'an informed scepticism for the claims made for it', quoting Green and others. Yet Knox was cautious because he thought the evidence was incomplete, not because he thought CIS was unimportant. The evidence at the time, he wrote, was 'compatible with the hypothesis that [CIS] *usually* [emphasis in original] progresses after a mean latent period of about ten years'. In particular he worried that the preinvasive stage was sometimes not long enough to be detected by screening. Nor did he foresee a study such as Green's as a realistic possibility: if women had CIS, treatment should be given.[19]

In the end all these men became convinced of the benefits of cervical screening based on data from Canada, and from other emerging studies, especially in the Nordic countries, which were brought together and reported by Matti Hakama in 1982.[20] In 1978 Professor Doll wrote to Professor Hugh McLaren, in Birmingham, after modifying his early views: 'You can count on me for maximum support for cervical cytology screening programmes in the future.'[21] These and many other organised population screening studies have repeatedly confirmed the value of the Pap smear and form the basis of organised international cervical screening programmes today.[22]

Classifying cervical cancer – 'staging', according to the extent to which a cancer has invaded the cervix and spread through the body – assists clinicians to determine its management and the patient's prognosis, and to audit results. Various international groups, beginning with the Cancer Committee of the League of Nations in 1928 and continuing through to the Fédération Internationale de Gynécologie et Obstétrique (FIGO) today, have, on the basis of international advice, modified and improved the staging system. FIGO, a notably conservative committee, recommended the addition of CIS – 'Stage 0' – as a special category in 1950:[23] this could only have happened on the basis of an overwhelming international consensus on the significance of CIS.

The inclusion of CIS in the FIGO staging system, together with a lively debate staged at the American Gynecologic Society in 1952 between the great clinician/pathologists Arthur Hertig, Paul Younge and John McKelvey, virtually ended any doubts about the malignant potential of CIS.[24] McKelvey, who had earlier claimed that all cases of CIS progressed to cancer, took the negative side of the debate and, like Green later, focused on the difficulties in the histological interpretation of lesions, but at no point did he say CIS had no relation to invasive cancer. McKelvey visited NWH in 1958 and 1963 and possibly influenced Green's evolving view of the natural history of CIS.

In the responses to a 1952 questionnaire on CIS sent to 160 gynaecology, pathology and cytology authorities in the United States, there was general agreement that:

- Cancer *in-situ* is Stage 0 cervical cancer.
- Cancer *in-situ* is a preinvasive stage of genuine cervical cancer.
- Routine cytological study is the detection method of choice, to be confirmed later by biopsy … a significant group favoured treatment depending on age, emphasising more *conservative* [my emphasis] therapy (ring biopsy, electro-conisation or amputation of the cervix).[25]

The only controversy concerned spontaneous regression, although most had never observed it. The majority favoured treatment, but some thought surgery should be withheld 'in order to determine behaviour and prove or disprove regression'.

* * *

By the mid-1960s there was almost universal acceptance of the view that cervical cancer developed from a precursor lesion – CIS.

In 1961 Dr Per Kolstad from Oslo compiled a table of clinical studies for the Norwegian Medical Society on the development of invasive cancer in untreated cases of CIS. He included 595 cases, from a number of reputable centres, followed from one to 23 years. In this large group 28 per cent developed cancer during follow-up.[26]

In 1963 Dr Leo Koss, one of Papanicolaou's protégés, reached the following conclusions as a result of a long-term study of cervical dysplasia and CIS:[27]

- carcinoma *in-situ* is a lesion of the cervical epithelium that beyond doubt is a precursor of cervical cancer
- carcinoma *in-situ* is very fragile and may be readily eradicated by a variety of minor procedures – such as small biopsies
- spontaneous disappearance of carcinoma *in-situ* apparently does occur, but it is an extraordinarily rare event
- histologically less advanced lesions classified as borderline atypias (dysplasias) behave similarly and may develop into carcinoma *in-situ* and even invasive cervical cancer
- carcinoma *in-situ* and lesser but related lesions have an extraordinarily slow evolution which continues over a period of many years.

There are limitations to all studies of the natural history of CIS. These include *method* – interference with the lesion through Pap smears and small diagnostic biopsies; *time* – the fact that the progression is best measured in decades, not years, and few studies extend this long; and *ethical issues* – best illustrated by the 'unfortunate experiment' carried out in New Zealand.[28]

The wide range in the reported proportions of women with untreated carcinoma *in-situ* progressing to cancer reflects the differing lengths of follow-up and, in the early studies, the lack of uniformity in pathology interpretation and definition. At no time did anyone suggest CIS 'invariably' or 'inevitably' progressed to cancer, or regressed to normal. Overall, however, there was remarkable uniformity in the various studies, with 20–30 per cent of women with persistent CIS of the cervix, either untreated or inadequately treated, progressing to cancer over a period of 10–15 years, and a proportion regressing to normal.[29] There was near unanimous agreement that women typically presented with CIS (usually following an abnormal smear test) in their mid- to late thirties, and with cancer in their late forties.[30]

Knowledge about the nature of the precursor abnormality, CIS, was acquired over many years from the work of many investigators. CIS had all the microscopic features of cancer, but had yet to invade the healthy tissue below. It was, however, at the most severe end of the spectrum of precancerous abnormalities. Once invasion below the basement membrane of the epithelium had occurred, an invasive cancer existed that was capable of killing the patient.

New Zealand kept abreast of international opinion. Dr Jefcoate Harbutt, gynaecological cancer surgeon at NWH, discussed the origin of cervical cancer at the first New Zealand Congress of the London-based Royal College of Obstetricians and Gynaecologists in 1955. He said 'the late and clinically obvious stages of cervical cancer constitute only a limited period in the life history of the disease ... increasing [heed] should be paid to the preclinical stage of development' and that 'carcinoma *in-situ* is a slowly progressive disease ... the only question which arises is how radical treatment should be'.[31] The same year, senior medical staff at NWH unanimously approved the establishment of a specialist cervical cancer team under Dr Harbutt's control. The staff agreed to a policy that 'carcinoma *in-situ* should be treated by hysterectomy except in cases where it is desirable to conserve reproductive function, when amputation of cervix should be carried out'.[32] This was in line with international opinion of the time.

Although the possibilities of gynaecological cytology were first explored in New Zealand in 1947 by Dr Lindsay Brown, it was not until the appointment of Harvey Carey as professor in 1953 that cervical cytology developed as a discipline. It was at this time that Dr Stephen Williams, pathologist-in-charge at Greenlane Hospital, 'agreed reluctantly' to process and examine approximately 1000 cytology slides 'to get Carey off my back'.[33] To his surprise, after about 200 specimens, a smear containing abnormal cells was detected in a symptomless woman: this convinced Williams that cytology might have something to offer. New Zealand's first cervical cytology screening laboratory was established at NWH in 1954 and, according to Green, 'had a fair start on the rest of New Zealand, Australia and Britain'.[34] Dr Gabriele Medley, director of the Victorian Cytology Service 1987–2000, agreed, noting that in the early days Australian cytotechnologists came to train at NWH.[35]

In 1955 Dr John Sullivan, a pathologist with an interest in smear tests and precancer, was appointed to NWH. In 1957 he studied cytology in Chicago with Dr George Wied who, like Koss, was a student of Papanicolaou. On his return to New Zealand he reported to the senior medical staff that in the centres he had recently visited in the United States 'there is now almost universal agreement that invasive carcinoma is at all sites preceded by an histologically recognisable *in-situ* stage' and that 'the majority of, if not all, invasive cervical cancers are preceded by a preinvasive stage'.[36]

In 1958 Carey and Williams reported 'surprise positives' in 2.4 per cent of gynaecological patients and 3 per cent of obstetric patients.[37] The term they used to describe the finding of malignant cells in a smear beautifully illustrated the excitement arising from this new precancer detection technique. In the same year Carey reported to the Auckland Hospital Board that during a three-year cytology survey, 20,000 smears had been taken and the lives of 40 women had been saved at a cost of £170 each.[38]

When Green arrived at NWH in 1956 he was nicely positioned to take advantage of the knowledge that CIS was a cancer precursor, and of the benefits to be derived from the recently introduced technique of cervical screening. His stated aim, 'to seek a means by which this particular type of cancer could be prevented', was within his grasp; thousands of New Zealand women would benefit; he could report his findings to the world and receive plaudits.[39]

* * *

While knowledge concerning the natural history of carcinoma *in-situ* accrued slowly over the first half of the 20th century, treatment of CIS became an issue only when the numbers of detected cases began to increase following the introduction of the cervical smear test in the 1950s. At this time conventional management was total hysterectomy, including the cervix. The few surgeons who regarded CIS as an early form of cancer performed radical hysterectomy, which included removal of the uterus, fallopian tubes, ovaries, upper vagina and pelvic lymph nodes. However, in 1958 the Hospital Medical Committee at NWH determined that, in accordance with an international trend,[40] the 'official hospital policy regarding the treatment of carcinoma of the cervix stage 0 [CIS] should [now] be adequate cone biopsy provided the immediate follow-up is negative and … the pathologist is satisfied the cone biopsy has included *all* [my emphasis] the carcinomatous material'.[41] The object of the treatment was to be the complete eradication of CIS, using a conservative method in order to retain the uterus.

Hysterectomy remained the generally preferred treatment in New Zealand hospitals other than NWH until the mid-1960s, when the 'new' conservative local treatments such as cone biopsy and amputation of the cervix were introduced, particularly for the increasing numbers of young women with the condition. Green must be given credit for introducing the new fertility-sparing cone biopsy into New Zealand: he was following less radical techniques that had been developed overseas a decade earlier. Cone biopsies involve cone-shaped pieces of tissue being excised from the cervix, including at least 2cm of the lower canal. The intention is to remove the CIS lesion in its entirety, but since the surgeon is unable to see the extent of the abnormality with the naked eye, complete excision is a hit-and-miss affair. Green later became an enthusiast for a smaller cone biopsy, the 'ring biopsy', which contained less than 2cm of cervical canal – this provided him with adequate tissue for diagnosis, the exclusion of cancer, although 'while it may completely excise the lesion [carcinoma in-situ] it cannot be considered definitive therapy'.[42] As a result some women continued to have abnormal smears following ring biopsy.[43]

Green's early lecture notes recorded his view at that stage on the nature and treatment of CIS. In 1957 he said CIS was 'nearly always found at the edge of a frank carcinoma ... many cases are on record in which carcinoma in-situ has progressed to cancer in times varying between one and 13 years'. He also reported a 1949 case at NWH in which CIS was found incidentally during a biopsy: three years later the woman concerned had developed cancer. He went on to say, '[T]he evidence seems almost certain that preinvasive cancer if left untreated will progress to invasive cancer. Exceptionally, some cases may regress. If it is not important to retain childbearing function total hysterectomy is the best treatment.'[44]

Two years later his lecture notes reflected an evolution in his thinking, in line with progressive international opinion: 'carcinoma in-situ is a [pre] cancer which can be eradicated 100% effectively ... hysterectomy is not an absolute therapeutic necessity ... treatment can be individualised ... hysterectomy can be preserved for those with persistent abnormal smears ...'[45] In 1962 Green's first published paper on CIS discussed the 'new' conservative management, concluding it was 'without risk to the patient'.[46] His lecture notes displayed his detailed examination of the international literature; he pointed out variations in pathology interpretation, the limitations of small 'diagnostic' biopsies and, quoting Krieger, stated 'it is likely, on tenuous grounds, a great number of women have been simultaneously subjected to hysterectomy, and psychologically traumatised by the fear of cancer'.[47]

One hundred and thirty doctors attended the first New Zealand Cancer Conference held at NWH in 1959 under the auspices of the New Zealand branch of the British Empire Cancer Campaign, with Dr George Wied of Chicago as the guest speaker. It was at this conference, which served as a catalyst for the wider use of cytology in New Zealand, that Wied suggested New Zealand should start a national cervical screening programme, an event that did not take place until three decades later, on the recommendation of the Cartwright Inquiry.[48]

At the 1959 conference, Dr Green, a young academic obstetrician and gynaecologist, was reported in the *Auckland Star* as saying:

> *Thanks to modern diagnostic techniques [cervical smears] an increasing number of cases of cervical cancer [he meant CIS] are now discovered so early that 100% cures are possible in precancer found in this way, before any clinical symptoms are present …*

> *Treatment could often consist of simple local surgery instead of removal of the uterus, because smears taken after treatment would immediately reveal any recurrence of the disease, or incomplete treatment …*

> *If undiscovered or left undetected, a third of these 'cancers' [CIS] would spread and be more difficult to treat within 9 years.*[49]

These statements fitted with the international opinion of the time that about one-third of cases of CIS would eventually progress to invasive cancer. And yet by 1966, Green was experimenting with merely observing cases of CIS following a small diagnostic biopsy. His views were undergoing radical change.

* * *

The third important figure in this story enters at this time. William McIndoe was known to all as Bill. Born in Auckland, the son of a tradesman engineer, he left Auckland Grammar School during the latter part of the Great Depression and began an electrical apprenticeship. Feeling the need for more intellectual stimulation he completed, part time, a Bachelor of Science majoring in physics, at Auckland University.

When the war broke out his skills saw him employed in the radar division of the Department of Scientific and Industrial Research. Later he transferred to the army and married his Bible class sweetheart, Noeline, on his final leave. After the war he entered Otago Medical School, assisted financially by a philanthropic member of the Roslyn Presbyterian Church, and graduated in 1950. He then spent two years as a house surgeon in Dunedin Hospital, followed by a year as a pathology registrar in Palmerston North. For four years he worked as a general practitioner in Hawera but found the role of a country doctor without obstetric experience to be lonely, frustrating and unfulfilling, so he decided to specialise in obstetrics and gynaecology. This necessitated a move to NWH as a 40-year-old trainee registrar, during which time he worked for Herb Green, who was of similar age and had recently joined the senior medical staff.

McIndoe was a kindly, unremarkable, compassionate gentleman. Beneath his reserved and self-effacing manner lay a strongly principled, sharp, analytical mind and a warm sense of humour. His deep Christian conviction led to his role as a session clerk in his local Presbyterian church, he was a regular runner with the church harriers, and he sang with the Auckland Choral Society. Despite his reserved nature he related easily to everyone, irrespective of their station in life. He viewed patients as equals, rarely referring to them as Miss, or Mrs, but simply as 'Sunshine' – he always called me 'Ronnie, my boy'.

One of McIndoe's ward sisters described him as 'humble, intelligent and a good communicator', but with colleagues he often appeared diffident and apologetic. While McIndoe was conservative by nature, he was sufficiently liberal to see the perspectives of others: he told me that in the early years of Green's experiment he acknowledged that Green might even have a point: the slow rate of progression of carcinoma *in-situ* to cancer meant that, in the initial period, very few women with persisting CIS did develop cancer. Serendipity had positioned McIndoe in the university of life, preparing him for the unknown challenge that lay ahead – dealing with Green's unnecessary and unfortunate experiment.

McIndoe sailed for England in 1961, working his passage as a ship's doctor for the princely sum of one shilling. He left his wife and family in New Zealand because there were insufficient funds. There he passed the membership examination for the Royal College of Obstetricians and Gynaecologists, then spent a year broadening his clinical experience, including further study of cervical cytology. Cervical cytology was a newly emerging field and McIndoe used his spare time to refine the skills he had begun to learn as a pathology registrar. Like Green, he wrote his thesis on the place of cytology in the prevention of cervical cancer.

He returned to New Zealand and was appointed to a part-time visiting obstetrician and gynaecologist position at NWH, with a subspecialty focus in cytology: his contract did not include major surgery. During this time he reported on a pilot community study, initiated by Professor Carey, of cervical screening in the Thames area.[50] He was keen to learn more about the emerging technique of colposcopy.

Colposcopy involves the use of a microscope to improve direct examination of the cervix. In 1960, following a visit by Austrian gynaecologist Professor Ernst Navratil, the hospital purchased a colposcope, which remained unused until McIndoe showed an interest in it. To begin with, McIndoe used pre-war German textbooks to teach himself but, realising the limitations of this, he went to Sydney in 1963 and spent three months with Dr Malcolm Coppleson, an early authority on the subject.

Colposcopy was first developed in Germany in the 1920s and 1930s, in the era before cervical smears, as a means of screening for and detecting microscopic cancers invisible to the naked eye. Following the development of the Pap smear, colposcopy came to be used for more detailed examination of the cervix in women with abnormal smears. A handful of doctors, including Adolf Stafl from Czechoslovakia and the US, James MacLean from Argentina, Per Kolstad from Oslo, Rene Cartier from Paris and Malcolm Coppleson from Sydney, were at the forefront of this 'new' colposcopy. McIndoe became friends with all these men, corresponded with them and visited their clinics: through him I was introduced to them all.

McIndoe remained a lifelong student of colposcopy, honing his skills, presenting papers at international conferences and, at Coppleson's request, providing him with photographs for his textbooks.[51] Coppleson always viewed carcinoma *in-situ* as a cancer precursor – a condition requiring complete eradication.[52] For the next decade, McIndoe was New Zealand's only colposcopist, running clinics at NWH and privately, and later practising and teaching the technique at major North Island centres. In 1974 he was elected a Member of the International Academy of Cytology.

* * *

In the mid-1960s Green's view on the nature of CIS evolved further. Having once regarded it as a precancerous condition, he now saw it as relatively benign. At this time he met, and was influenced by, the studies of a Perth gynaecologist, Dr Ellis Pixley. Pixley was an alternative thinker, though not in the academic mould, who had studied the cervices of stillborn girls, early perinatal deaths and those of young children who had died in accidents. He told Green he had noted similar microscopic appearances in these cervices to those seen in the cervices of women with precancerous changes. Later Green said, 'Around 1963 I thought that the abnormal cytology in women developing carcinoma *in-situ* or cancer may have been present since birth: this was because many pathologists and clinicians I consulted diagnosed dysplasia or carcinoma *in-situ* in autopsy specimens of the cervices of stillborn infants.'[53]

Green decided to replicate Pixley's study and examine tissue samples from the cervices of female stillbirths and neonatal deaths. In the 1965 annual report of the Postgraduate School of Obstetrics and Gynaecology he wrote: 'The histology of some 200 foetal cervices has commenced. Several have revealed epithelial dysplasia bearing a strong resemblance to adult lesions.' In the next report, Green noted that he was studying 'the morphology and histology of the pre-pubertal cervix [which] gives some promise of elucidating the natural history of the disease'. He acknowledged this work was being done in collaboration with Pixley. The following year he reported that 'many macroscopic and microscopic features found in the foetal cervix have their counterpart in the adult cervix but in the latter connotation are regarded as abnormal'.[54]

In another study on this topic he organised nursing staff to collect samples of vaginal cells, taken with small swabs, from healthy newborn girls, to test for abnormal cells. These tests were performed without the knowledge of the mothers.

Herb Green took a keen interest in the microscopic assessment (histopathology) of cervical CIS and cancer; this followed the path already established by cancer surgeons elsewhere, including one of his mentors, Dr Stanley Way in Gateshead, Newcastle. Green had no formal pathology training, but rather 'picked it up' when reviewing cases with trained pathology colleagues such as John Sullivan, Jim Gwynne, Jock McLean and overseas specialists.

Michael Churchouse, a diminutive, likeable, uncomplicated man, was appointed charge technologist in the NWH Cytology Laboratory in 1962; this placed him in an ideal position to view Green's influence on cytology. Regarding Green's later claim at the Cartwright Inquiry that 'he had only done about 200 smears [on newborn baby girls] and they were for gonorrhoea checks', Churchouse noted that these were 'taken by "cotton tipped applicators" from the vagina' and were 'wet fixed, only suitable for cytological examination, and not suitable for bacterial examination'. Churchouse recorded:

> This so-called short-term study went from late 1963 and tapered off only in 1966 when it finally stopped. The '200' smears stretched to 2244 baby smears. The incredible reason for this study was Prof Green's vague belief that perhaps he could surprise the world with a finding of early cancer in neonates. As regards to this finding he was quite wrong, they were all negative.

> The screeners, all young women, were quite rebellious and critical of having to put our heavy workload to one side to screen these smears which they felt were immoral and routinely taken without the mothers' permission. An added spur to the staff's rage was that one of our recently retired staff was about to enter the ward to give birth, and there was nothing left unsaid as to what the staff would do if her name appeared on a baby smear. Luckily this did not happen but nevertheless with the staff behind me we made a general complaint to our pathologist, Dr Darby, who decided he would screen all the baby slides himself.[55]

Green did not report the findings of the vaginal smear or cervix tissue studies, despite the human and economic toll, presumably because no abnormalities were detected. If he had 'confirmed' his hypothesis he surely would have published such ground-breaking research in order to provide further scientific validity. He did, however, provide a photograph for Coppleson's textbook.[56] Pixley published his findings a decade later when he and others reported that the infant cervix tissue represented normal developmental changes.[57] Green's comments on his observations of the fetal cervix provide a foundation for the evolution of his views on the nature of CIS of the cervix. In the 1968 annual report, he wrote: '[T]he relatively benign nature of so-called "carcinoma *in-situ*" has now been established with confirmation from studies of fetal and neonatal cervices from necropsy material.'[58]

Green's early observations led him to believe in what he termed 'dormant' cancer. Many years later two patients appearing at the Cartwright Inquiry reported comments Green made to them. One woman said he told her, 'Nine out of 10 women have cancer … and … in cases like that, it lies dormant.' The other said Green told her 'every person is normally born with cancer, but it is the type of cancer that is dormant ... sometimes it just flares up'.[59] It seems likely that Green deduced the adult lesion was less dangerous than conventional gynaecology deemed it to be, since the microscopic findings in the fetus or newborn did not develop into cancer in childhood or early adult life.

It is possible he considered immunological factors might play a role in preventing the progression of CIS to cancer. He would have been familiar with the evolving evidence of the immunological relationship between a mother and her fetus and, no doubt, he would have observed the regression of CIS during pregnancy or following a tiny biopsy. Later he began research in cancer immunology.

* * *

Cone biopsy, Green's second phase of 'conventional' CIS management, lasted from 1958 to mid-1965. A 1964 paper revealed a further evolution in his thinking: '[C]arcinoma *in-situ* is probably benign in the great majority of cases.'[60] This led to Green's third management phase, officially from 1966 (but starting earlier): punch biopsy without definitive treatment – the 'unfortunate experiment'. The same year he had also begun to observe, but not treat, women with vulval and vaginal CIS. In 1965 he had said 'the series is unique in the world'.[61]

Thus, over a seven-year period, Green's opinion evolved from the orthodox view of CIS being 'almost certain[ly]' a precancer to its being 'probably benign'.

His iconoclastic views were being challenged by experts beyond New Zealand before his 1966 study began. At a seminar on the 'Diagnosis of carcinoma *in-situ*', sponsored by the Anti-Cancer Council of South Australia in July 1965, Green presented a paper on 'The significance of carcinoma *in-situ*', and Dr James Kirkland, an Adelaide pathologist, presented two papers on the subject – 'The pathology of carcinoma *in-situ* and early invasive carcinoma' and 'The chromosomal and mitotic abnormalities in preinvasive and invasive carcinomas of the cervix'.[62] Margaret Stanley, Professor of Epithelial Cell Biology at Cambridge University, met both men at this seminar. She vividly recalled Kirkland arguing forcibly with Green, pointing out that pathological and cytological evidence overwhelmingly demonstrated that CIS and invasive cancer were part of the same spectrum of neoplastic disease, the only difference being that CIS had yet to invade the underlying tissue and threaten the life of the woman.

Green dismissed Kirkland's scientific views.[63] He had begun to believe that CIS and cervical cancer were in fact different diseases. And from about 1963 he had begun to formulate in his mind a study of the natural history of CIS of the cervix, involving the observation of a large group of women, without definitive treatment.

Dr Albert Singer, now Professor of Obstetrics and Gynaecology at the University of London, was a registrar at the King George V Hospital in Sydney when Green visited Coppleson's colposcopy clinic in 1966. There was 'animated discussion' leading to 'strong language' when Coppleson refused to support Green in his forthcoming study.[64]

Both Coppleson and Kirkland had strong personalities and both had attained national and international reputations as authorities on the natural history of CIS. Green was still only a big fish in a small New Zealand pond, yet to make his controversial views recognised in the wider international community. British epidemiologist Professor Jocelyn Chamberlain recalled that Green had visited Dr Max Wilson, author of the influential *Principles and Practice of Screening* and an early supporter of cervical screening in Britain. When Green told Wilson about his plans, the response was: 'that's fine so long as you do it as a randomised controlled trial comparing an untreated group with a treated group as the controls, with stopping rules, and a data-monitoring committee so that everything is above board.'[65]

As we will see, in Green's forthcoming experiment he had no control group, no stopping rules and no data-monitoring committee.

* * *

On 14 February 1964 NWH moved into a new, state-of-the art, multistorey building in a pleasant, parklike setting. This was now a true 'National' Women's Hospital, receiving difficult and challenging obstetric and gynaecological cases from all over New Zealand. The latest in patient care was available, and student and postgraduate teaching equalled the best in the world. The hospital was buzzing with the excitement of its research, including the world's first successful intrauterine transfusion for rhesus disease performed by Professor Bill Liley the previous year.[66] As Sir Douglas Robb observed, 'The young medical men … are in full cry. They ask to be judged by nothing less than world standards, and if we can feed them the opportunities, the equipment and the resources they need, they will soon have us thoroughly on the world map of medicine.'[67]

From the 1960s through to the 1980s, NWH functioned as two separate units. In the university department, 'A' Team was responsible for teaching, research and a proportion of daily clinical duties, and 'D' Team for the management of women with cervical cancer. Clinical duties were shared with the non-academic 'B' and 'C' Teams, which consisted mainly of part-time visiting specialist obstetricians and gynaecologists.

Patients usually remained under the care of the consultant who had first seen them at the hospital, and his team. Bonham was head of the university department, and Green, Liley and Liggins were responsible to him. A medical hierarchy existed, not only within the membership of individual teams – usually as a function of seniority – but also between the teams. Dr Kevin Hill remembered a confrontation in the surgeons' change room between a fellow registrar, Dr Paul Hutchison, and Bonham, who took strong exception to Hutchison referring to him simply as 'Prof', and not 'Professor'. Hutchison, in his own defence, replied that he had used the word as a term of endearment. Bonham retorted, 'You are only fit to work on B team!' Not only was this a put-down for Hutchison, but also for the non-academic members on B and C team: on this assessment I was the lowermost member of the lowermost clinical team in the hospital.[68]

The non-academic medical teams were responsible, through the medical superintendent and the overall medical superintendent-in-chief, to the Auckland Hospital Board. Links between the teams were provided by Jock McLean, who performed histopathology, and Bill McIndoe, who, with other cytopathologists, was responsible for cytology and colposcopy. Jefcoate Harbutt and later Liam Wright were the visiting D team cervical cancer surgeons.

The Senior Medical Staff Committee and the Hospital Medical Committee were responsible for the medical administration of NWH. The former, chaired by the medical superintendent, was a forum where all hospital specialists could discuss medical matters. The latter had been established by the Hospitals Amendment Act 1947 to oversee the clinical organisation of NWH. It had a de facto responsibility for research and ethics within both the hospital and the university department. Its membership was established by statute. The Hospitals Act 1957 stated that the postgraduate professor, and not the medical superintendent, should chair the Hospital Medical

Committee. This was a festering sore for non-university senior medical staff, who made up the bulk of the hospital staff. Green and Bonham, who was the committee's chair for most of this period, opposed change for many years. The act was finally changed in 1978 and the medical superintendent became chair of the Hospital Medical Committee.

The Hospital Medical Committee comprised a limited group of senior academics, full-time specialists and senior medical staff. It received advice from the Senior Medical Staff Committee and had executive and de facto ethics committee roles. Senior medical staff who were not members of the Hospital Medical Committee considered it to be undemocratic; this was the basis for much frustration. Dr John Stewart, full-time charge radiologist, and McLean, pathologist-in-charge, both told me they were conscious that their opinions were not valued by the Hospital Medical Committee hierarchy. Some junior specialist members of the NWH deliberately avoided involvement in hospital politics.

The scene was now set for these two committees to determine whether Associate Professor Green should proceed with a formal proposal to observe women with CIS of the cervix without definitive treatment.

CHAPTER 3

AN UNNECESSARY EXPERIMENT

... a woman with [CIS] lives under the sword of Damocles. It may never
strike but the risk of it doing so increases with each passing year.

JOHN STALLWORTHY, 1966[1]

IN 1966 MY WIFE Barbara, baby daughter Helen and I began the most
important journey in our lives – a five-week sea trip to England to enable
me to begin my postgraduate studies. We were away for over six years,
during which time I passed the FRCS (surgery) and MRCOG (obstetrics
and gynaecology) examinations. I came back to the tutor specialist position
at NWH in 1973.

1966 was also the year Professor Herbert Green sought approval for
a study that involved observing a large group of women with CIS of the
cervix, without definitive treatment, and without their consent. Ideally
he would have liked a multi-centre study, but as most New Zealand
gynaecologists still treated CIS with hysterectomy there was little point in
inviting them to participate. His only potential ally, Coppleson in Sydney,
who was eradicating CIS conservatively with cone biopsy, had declined
Green's invitation to take part. Green had no choice but to do the study
himself at NWH. He recognised that the proposed study was a significant
departure from the agreed hospital treatment policy and he would therefore
need the approval of the hospital authorities. These were the days before
the establishment of ethics committees but in some respects NWH was
ahead of its time in requiring its Hospital Medical Committee to approve
any changes of policy or procedure, and Green's study was a significant
departure from the 1958 policy of cone biopsy.

Was Green equipped to perform a study with such far-reaching
consequences? He had no formal training in clinical research; he had
no mentor; he had not worked in a recognised academic unit beyond
the nascent NWH. In Green's defence, as Professor Barbara Heslop later

pointed out, research at that time was 'all about some of the ignorance and naivety of a previous age … when clinical research was relatively unsophisticated and unstructured'.[2] Green had no protocol; he worked alone – not as part of a multidisciplinary team, as happens today. He was arrogant and believed he knew more than those around him. Although he did not clearly enunciate an hypothesis, the minutes of the 1966 meeting that approved his study stated: '[H]is aim is to attempt to prove that carcinoma in-situ is not a premalignant disease.'[3] Green perhaps did not understand that an hypothesis needs to be falsifiable. His aim of proving that CIS did not lead to invasive cancer would have been falsified once the first cases of cancer occurred.

In early June 1966 Green's formal written proposal was circulated with the agendas for the forthcoming Senior Medical Staff Committee and Hospital Medical Committee meetings.[4] Bill McIndoe read the proposal with trepidation: he knew all the medical staff believed CIS was a precancer and therefore treated it, but sensed that out of loyalty to 'a Kiwi doing research' they might go along with Green's proposal.[5] He wrote 'a memorandum of comment on Green's suggestions' and decided to discuss his concerns with Bruce Grieve, one of the hospital's most senior and respected gynaecologists. Grieve was an intelligent, straightforward man with a strong personality – a natural leader. He had a particular interest in gynaecological pathology, later chairing the Hospital Tumour Panel from its inception in 1971 until his retirement in 1976. McIndoe reported that Grieve 'heard me patiently but indicated that he felt prepared to allow Professor Green to proceed'. McIndoe also discussed his memorandum with Algar Warren, the medical superintendent, and on the advice of both men he removed the final sentence: 'If Professor Green's proposal is accepted I would feel it very difficult to take seriously any cytology reporting or colposcopy assessment.'[6]

On 20 June 1966, a cold, midwinter evening, Green submitted a poorly constructed proposal – 'to attempt to prove that carcinoma in-situ is not a premalignant disease' – to the meetings of the Senior Medical Staff Committee and later the Hospital Medical Committee.[7] In support of his proposal Green provided evidence from his existing study of women with CIS of the cervix. He stated that only one of 503 women with CIS managed in NWH from 1946 to 1966 had developed cancer, a figure approximating the expected incidence in the general population. The minutes of the Senior Medical Staff Committee meeting did not reveal Green's failure to emphasise that nearly all these women had been treated, and as a result few, if any, would have been expected to develop cancer. He also said he was currently monitoring eight cases of patients with continuing smear abnormalities who had not had a cone or ring biopsy: his experiment was clearly under way. Yet four years earlier, his trusted pathologist, Sullivan, had reported at an international meeting that three cases of invasive cancer had developed among 126 women treated for CIS; he also predicted that 'the true number of cases will certainly be much higher'.[8] There is no evidence in the minutes whether Green referred to the overwhelming international view that CIS did, in a proportion of cases, progress to cancer, or quoted reported rates of progression.

Green later paraphrased the lengthy, and in part obscure, minutes of the motion passed by the Hospital Medical Committee: 'In 1965 [sic] the senior medical staff of NWH initiated a project under the supervision of the author, for patients up to 35 years of age whose only abnormal finding was positive cervical cytology … Providing the [diagnostic] punch biopsy did not remove the entire significant area, or reveal invasive cancer, there was to be no further [sic] treatment'.[9] Women with a known premalignant condition were to be observed without treatment – and without their knowledge or consent. The stenographer responsible for taking the minutes of the meeting recorded that 'in the interests of continuity and patient confidence, it is suggested all cases should be passed to the care of Professor Green, whose conscience is clear and who can therefore accept complete responsibility for whatever happens'.[10]

Bill McIndoe presented his written memorandum to this meeting and expressed his concerns about Green's proposed study. He did not address the later Hospital Medical Committee meeting because he was not a member. However, he provided a written statement that clearly set out his views.

He began by acknowledging that Green had 'made an important contribution to the treatment of carcinoma *in-situ* of the cervix in his insistence on less radical care and his claim that local excision and follow-up is adequate treatment. Initially … cone biopsy seemed a reasonable measure'. Now, however, colposcopy meant that the area of concern could usually be identified and the right type of excision used.

Again, I believe Professor Green has made a useful contribution in insisting … progression from in-situ *to invasive carcinoma of the cervix is not invariable. I do, however, find it difficult to accept his statement that carcinoma* in-situ *and invasive carcinoma of the cervix are not related conditions. On morphological grounds the appearance of the cells, in dysplasia, carcinoma* in-situ *and invasive carcinoma of the cervix there does seem to be a relationship.*

McIndoe accepted that progression from CIS to cancer 'may be uncommon' but 'At our present state of knowledge rather than swing to an extremely conservative position with respect to treatment, I feel the correct measure would be to aim to remove tissue responsible for the positive smear and to follow up patients conservatively thereafter who show no further significant cytological or colposcopic abnormality.' He went on to say:

Furthermore, I believe an authoritative approach to any problem in medicine can be unfortunate unless it is quite obvious alternative methods of care are either dangerous or unsound. In the present case inadequate tissue diagnosis, which can be the only description of the type of biopsy [punch] I at present perform (if this is to be the only biopsy done) and follow-up only taking further steps if there is clinical or colposcopic evidence of invasion, would seem to me the type of care which should not be followed. Conservative excision of the lesion is in my view the treatment of choice.[11]

At the Cartwright Inquiry 18 years later a number of senior doctors, including Green, Bonham, Grieve and Bruce Faris, could not recall McIndoe tabling or speaking to the memorandum,[12] but Warren, the medical superintendent, clearly remembered the occasion, and McIndoe visiting him the next day, concerned he had not expressed his position strongly enough. McIndoe referred to his 1966 memorandum again in 1973, when he reiterated the point in further memoranda.

There was extensive discussion at the 1966 Senior Medical Staff Committee meeting about Green's proposed research, including the provision of a number of safeguards: the study would be limited to women under 35 years, and cancer was to be excluded at the outset using Green's expertise and colposcopic examinations by McIndoe. The minutes of the meeting recorded: 'If at any stage concern is felt for the safety of the patient, a cone biopsy is to be performed.'[13]

The only inference that can be drawn from the words 'concern' and 'safety of the patient' is that a cancer might already be present or might develop; after all, CIS is at the serious end of the spectrum of cervical precancer. No one except McIndoe appeared to appreciate that there was no safety barrier. If cancer was present it was already too late; if a woman had CIS, a symptomless microscopic condition, there was a risk of cancer, with its attendant morbidity and mortality. Professor Mont Liggins, writing in 2003, put it succinctly: 'It was an experiment with two possible end points – invasive cancer or no invasive cancer. This did not occur to Green.'[14] Note Liggins' use of the word 'experiment'.

The Senior Medical Staff meeting of 20 June 1966 was long, finishing shortly before 9pm, when the meeting of the Hospital Medical Committee, the body responsible for approving research projects, began. There was a long agenda – 11 items in all. The item preceding the confirmation of Green's proposal had an obstetric flavour: following a proposal by Harbutt it was resolved that 'When the patient wants her husband to be notified of the birth, a reasonable attempt should be made to contact him by phone and the Board be requested to provide telephones in every delivery theatre.'[15]

Item nine was Green's proposal. All 11 members of the Hospital Medical Committee – Bonham (chair), Warren, Alastair Macfarlane, Grieve, Harbutt, Green, Faris, Ian Hutchison, Jack Matthews, John Stewart and McLean – had been present at the earlier meeting and would have been familiar with the discussion. The minutes of the Senior Medical Staff meeting record 'a lengthy discussion during which Professor Green answered many questions', but the brevity of the minutes on this item at the later meeting suggests that the Hospital Medical Committee simply 'rubber stamped' Green's proposal without further consideration.[16]

The men who moved and seconded the motion to approve Green's experiment were both trusted and well liked. Surprisingly, it was the hospital's youthful radiologist, Dr John Stewart, who put the motion; his experience and discipline did not equip him to consider the long-term consequences of Green's study. Senior gynaecologist Alastair Macfarlane, who seconded the motion, also clearly failed to recognise the potential sequelae of the experiment. However, both he and fellow senior gynaecologist, Grieve, despite voting for Green's proposal, said they did not wish to transfer their patients to Green's study, preferring to care for (i.e. treat) them themselves. There can be only two possible explanations for their ambiguous decisions:

either they lacked confidence in Green's hypothesis or, in their roles as well-known private practitioners, they did not wish to be seen to be supporting him publicly.

* * *

Why was the proposal accepted? There was a well-established medical hierarchy within the hospital, with academic members of the postgraduate school at the top and non-academic medical specialists making up the bulk of the staff. In matters of research the latter deferred to the academics, whose role included the critical examination of scientific evidence. It is not surprising that when McIndoe, a quietly spoken doctor at the bottom of the pecking order, spoke out against Green's proposal, his opinion was taken less seriously than it should have been. As lawyer Hugh Rennie, counsel for McIndoe's estate, stated later at the Cartwright Inquiry, it was 'equivalent to the office boy trying to tell the managing director how to run the firm'.[17] And of course McIndoe, unlike Green, was not a member of the Hospital Medical Committee, which gave final approval for the study to proceed.

Herb Green, an associate professor, was trusted by his colleagues, and there was likely to have been an element of sympathy for him because he missed out on the postgraduate chair. Finally, human nature being what it is, there may have been little interest in his academic proposal – it was late in the day and the clinical staff would have been anxious to get home. The way was now clear: the proposal had been approved. Green could forge ahead, accumulate as many cases as he could and report his results to the medical world. Despite his reservations about the study, McIndoe did initially provide colposcopic assistance.

Did Green's research constitute an experiment? He himself did not use the word 'experiment' to describe his work. He called it a 'study', a 'project', a 'special series'. The word 'experiment' was not applied to Green's study until almost two decades after its inception, when Professor David Skegg referred to 'the unfortunate experiment'. Skegg said that

> in epidemiology and clinical studies of humans there are two broad kinds of investigation: observational studies and experimental studies. The fundamental difference is that in an experiment the conditions are under the direct control of the investigators. They do not merely observe what is going on, but can intervene – such as the administration of a new treatment or (less commonly) the withholding of conventional treatment.[18]

Skegg had no doubt that Green was conducting an experiment, and the Cartwright Inquiry Report subsequently agreed.

* * *

Thus from 1966 there were two quite separate and parallel management policies at NWH for women with CIS of the cervix. One set of women consisted largely of private patients referred to the hospital by a specialist member of the visiting staff on B and C teams, and managed by them. These women received conventional treatment as described by Green in his 1968 lecture notes for postgraduate doctors. He stated that 'conventional treatment comprises: (a) cone biopsy excision ... a certain proportion [will] continue to have doubtful or positive smears in the follow-up period ... and require further biopsy excision or even hysterectomy [as previously defined in the 1958 hospital protocol] and (b) hysterectomy'.[19] In this set of women, the aim was to eradicate CIS with a view to normal follow-up smears.

A second set were women with smear abnormalities who were referred by their general practitioners to the public clinic at NWH and were directed to Green's D team – 'all such cases should be passed to the care of Professor Green'.[20] Green stated that 'providing the [diagnostic] biopsy did not remove the entire significant area or reveal invasive carcimoma, there was to be no further [sic] treatment'.[21] Many women would continue to have smear abnormalities and be followed indefinitely in Green's clinic, unknowingly becoming part of the 'unfortunate experiment'. These statements by Green provide evidence of two simultaneous and different management policies at NWH for CIS of the cervix:

• 'Conventional' treatment by conisation or hysterectomy; or
• An experiment withholding definitive treatment (i.e. observing) the CIS.

General practitioners who were aware of Green's experiment and who were not prepared to have their patients observed without treatment referred them, privately in the first instance, to a specialist on the visiting staff, who would then arrange treatment by his own team.

Having gained approval for his study, Green became a lone voice. While there was debate regarding the proportion of women with untreated or inadequately treated CIS that will progress to cancer, no one else in the world was prepared simply to observe the untreated or inadequately treated lesion indefinitely. Dr Joe Jordan, who travelled the world extensively in the 1970s during his tenure as president of the International Federation of Cervical Pathology and Colposcopy (IFCPC), noted, 'I can honestly say that in world colposcopy there was not a colposcopist who shared Green's views.'[22]

CHAPTER 4

EXPRESSIONS OF CONCERN

Professor Green is entitled to his opinion, but it must be realised the vast majority of world authorities do not share it.

Ed Giesen

ONCE THE PROPOSAL TO observe women with CIS of the cervix without definitive treatment had been accepted, Green had a free hand to proceed with the experiment in the way he wished. He had only the flimsiest protocol to adhere to or to guide him. He was a senior member of the academic department and though he nominally had to answer to Bonham, this was more in the breach than in the observance. No doubt, however, Bonham would have been pleased to have Green's publications on the departmental annual report required by the university; academic departments are expected to contribute to the international literature and are judged on their ability to do so.

From the beginning Green ignored the safety issues that had been set out in his proposal to the Hospital Medical Committee. Without further approval he included women over 35, some with microinvasive cervical cancer (a condition in which CIS has penetrated the basement membrane below the epithelium – the earliest form of invasive cancer), and women with vulval and vaginal CIS. His aim was to accumulate as many cases as possible of untreated or undertreated CIS, evidenced by persistent smear abnormalities and, rather than treat them, to follow them indefinitely. This would enable him to prove that CIS was 'probably benign in the great majority of cases'.[1]

Had his research to date actually convinced him none of the women was likely to develop cancer? We can but guess. Today's science is largely collaborative, and rarely pursued in isolation, but Green's experiment depended almost entirely on him. He required laboratory support and, ideally, assistance from McIndoe, who was expected to play a subservient role – the David to his Goliath. Green did not suffer fools gladly: this was his experiment and he did not rate McIndoe. This is amply demonstrated by a letter Green wrote to Bonham complaining that one of his patients 'had not seen a senior consultant with any knowledge of carcinoma *in-situ* for four years'. The records showed the woman had seen McIndoe on four occasions during this time.[2]

The next few years were Green's honeymoon period. Cases were collected, results were collated and written up in medical journals, and on the international stage Green spoke extensively of his findings.

In a major paper in the *American Journal of Obstetrics and Gynecology* in 1966 he had suggested the risk of women with untreated CIS developing cancer was 'much less than 10%'.[3] The following year, in Bangkok, he said that 'cervical carcinoma *in-situ* of the cervix is not of serious import', and that in 503 women with CIS in his series, progression *had not been recorded in a single instance*.[4] In a 1969 paper he reported that 'the recent [international] literature shows that about one-third of *in-situ* cancers progress to invasion in about 12–20 years', yet in his series to date only one of 539 cases had developed cancer. The 'invasive potentiality of the disease is low', he concluded, and the previous overemphasis was due to inaccurate pathology diagnoses – 'possibly because of either initial under-diagnosis of invasive cancer or later over-diagnosis of *in-situ* cancer'.[5] The obvious implication was that pathologists elsewhere in the world were in error. In this same paper he also stated: 'By commonly accepted standards many *in-situ* lesions [under my care] have been almost disdainfully undertreated'.[6]

As might be expected in someone who spent much of his day looking down a microscope, McIndoe was a meticulous man. From the beginning he carefully documented the data from all women in the hospital diagnosed with CIS, not just those under Green's care. He was ideally placed to do so because he performed colposcopy on all women with abnormal smears, including Green's patients, and read the follow-up smear tests. Many years later he recalled his response when, during a world study tour in 1968, he was asked to comment on Green's work: 'I was bound to state, as I believed then and do now, that [Green] is not presenting the evidence fairly and in fact is biased in his reporting of what is actually happening in this hospital'.[7] In discussion with McLean, the pathologist, McIndoe had become aware that Green, although untrained as a pathologist, was independently reviewing the histology slides of women in his series and in some instances was reclassifying the diagnoses.[8]

On Monday mornings, Green, cancer surgeon Harbutt (and later his successor, Dr Liam Wright), McIndoe and resident medical staff met in Ward 9, assessed women with cervical cancer and, where appropriate, inserted radium treatment. Following the theatre session on 14 April 1969 McIndoe asked Green why he was reclassifying the diagnoses in some women. McIndoe was concerned that some women originally classified in the patient records as having CIS were being reclassified as having invasive cancer at the outset and therefore ineligible for his study. Others, originally diagnosed with invasive cancer, were being reclassified as having CIS. McIndoe was suggesting that Green was retrospectively manipulating the data, a serious accusation: 'I find myself in a difficult position in this study,' he later wrote.[9] Green made it clear that McIndoe had no right to confront him with such questions – this was *his* study, not McIndoe's.

McIndoe documented his comments in a letter sent to Green the following day, generously offering two suggestions that might have helped to resolve the problem. The first was an open correspondence between Australasian authorities in the *Australia and New Zealand Journal of Obstetrics and Gynaecology*,[10] and the second was a clinical meeting with Dr Malcolm Coppleson from Sydney to discuss difficult and contentious cases. Green did not respond to McIndoe's letter, claiming at the Cartwright Inquiry that he did not receive it. In my view, this is highly unlikely. Because McIndoe was well down the pecking order, his views were of no consequence and it is possible Green consigned his letter to the wastepaper bin. If a meeting had been held, Green would almost certainly have refused to accept any opposing views anyway.

I have personally read pathology forms where Green had handwritten a revised diagnosis on patients' reports, changing 'carcinoma *in-situ*' to 'invasive carcinoma', or vice versa. Michael Churchouse also recalled Green removing 'ALERT' stickers from patients' cytology reports and writing changed diagnoses on the form.[11]

Bryan Trenwith, who in 1965 was a trainee pathology registrar, later described McIndoe:

Outside the department I frequently ran into Bill McIndoe who was the kindest Christian gentleman. He was at that stage under great pressure as he began to question the veracity of Herb's theory about carcinoma in-situ *being a separate disease from invasive cervical cancer, and he had dared to express his contrary opinion. Bill was a shy and diffident man who would whisper in the corridor about his latest altercation. He would look around furtively to avoid being caught by Herb for what might be interpreted as a conspiratorial conversation. The conflict seemed to take its toll on Bill.*[12]

* * *

Follow-up of patients was a crucial part of the study and Green's loyal support staff went to considerable lengths to locate the women involved. In his 1969 paper for the *International Journal of Gynaecology and Obstetrics* he recorded a 100 per cent follow-up. If a patient failed to make an appointment (usually six-monthly) or did not reply to an enquiry, she was visited by one of the hospital's medico-social workers. Green noted that local and national home-nursing, social and legal agencies were used to locate defaulting patients. He also observed that 'close follow-up [is] not mentally traumatic to patients; if the physician does not worry too much about the disease then neither will the patient'.[13]

Patient records, however, demonstrate that Green was prepared to instruct his clinical records staff to go to even greater lengths to follow the women. To find his 'lost' patients he used methods that today would be considered highly unethical in the context of a research proposal where follow-up was not for the benefit of the patient. The patients' medical records illustrate how his administrative staff would begin their search using telephone books, progress to electoral rolls, then use 'contact names' from hospital records including relatives, friends and sometimes ex-husbands. Letters were sent to public health nurses, the Social Welfare Department, the Housing Corporations of New Zealand and Australia, and hospitals in New Zealand and overseas which women had previously attended. A solicitor who had represented a woman in a divorce case was identified from a newspaper article, and obliged Green with the woman's contact details. Green used newspaper information from police cases as an excuse to write to the police for patient contact details – he went as far as contacting Scotland Yard. He contacted the women's workplaces, their husbands or partners. He even approached the school a woman's children had previously attended, hoping to get a forwarding address. Through the *New Zealand Medical Register* he located the wives of New Zealand doctors who were overseas. Following identification of one woman's car, a 'note was left on a window'.

Green wrote to patients cautioning them against treatment by other practitioners, and to GPs and specialist colleagues encouraging them to continue observation of CIS. He wrote to one patient who moved to Wellington:

> You have the condition (carcinoma in-situ) which many people have thought in the past might go on to true cancer but which we have now realised in this hospital is not so. Gynaecologists generally, outside Auckland, without the facilities of National Women's Hospital, are naturally inclined to view this condition more radically than we do here and so I warn you that any specialist you may go to may suggest further surgery is necessary.[14]

The Wellington gynaecologist to whom Green referred the patient told him the patient had now moved to Christchurch. Green responded, 'She may be lucky if she gets away from Christchurch intact. I think Hamish McCrostie would be the best person to refer her to – at least I know him well enough to reproach him if he wants to do a hysterectomy.'[15]

In a major paper in the *Journal of Obstetrics and Gynaecology of the British Commonwealth* in 1970, Green described 'follow-up observations of 75 patients with untreated or incompletely treated carcinoma *in-situ*'. Twenty-two had had only a diagnostic punch biopsy. All had 'shown evidence of persistent disease' as revealed by smear abnormalities.[16] Green reported that none of these women had developed cancer. When, in 1987, I was instructed by the Cartwright Inquiry to report on the outcome in these 75 cases, I found that one-quarter of these women had in fact developed cancer. A later review revealed that one-third of the women had developed cancer.[17]

In another 1970 paper the editor of the *Australia and New Zealand Journal of Obstetrics and Gynaecology* added the words 'An atypical viewpoint' to the title of a paper in which Green described one case of cancer developing in 576 women with CIS – exactly the frequency expected in a normal population.[18] (McIndoe's handwritten analysis of the paper notes three women who had developed cancer.[19]) In the same paper Green reiterated the object of his study:

> The only way to settle the question as to what happens to carcinoma in-situ is to follow adequately diagnosed but untreated lesions indefinitely. This is a theoretical impossibility because diagnosis is always treatment to an indeterminate degree. However, it is being attempted at National Women's Hospital by means of 2 series of cases. (i) A group of 27

women ... [with cervical carcinoma in-situ*] are being followed without
'treatment' ... (ii) A group of 5 women ... with evidence of vaginal
carcinoma* in-situ *... without treatment.*

He concluded that 'the patient with *in-situ* cancer has only the normal
chance of developing future invasive cancer'.[20]

The first thing to note is that Green here clearly indicates he is following
'adequately diagnosed but *untreated* lesions indefinitely'. Secondly, we, the
authors of the 1984 paper, have been criticised for 'grouping' patients for the
purpose of analysis. Yet here Green is himself grouping patients into those
with *cervical* CIS without treatment and those with *vaginal* CIS without
treatment. We might further note that Green was never given a mandate to
study women with vulval and vaginal CIS.

Green's publications were beginning to attract comment in the
international literature. J.P. Greenhill, the editor of the *1970 Year Book of
Obstetrics & Gynecology*, wrote: 'Green has repeatedly expressed his idea
preinvasive cervical carcinoma *in-situ* is not a significant lesion. He has
repeatedly written invasive carcinoma of the cervix will not eventually be
eliminated by cytological screening techniques. This is in direct contrast to
what most cytologists, pathologists and gynecologists believe.'[21]

In the same year, a paper by Green was used as a subject for debate by
a number of eminent American physicians. The debate was published in
Modern Medicine in the United States, but not in New Zealand. Green was
strongly condemned by some contributors. William Christopherson found
it 'incomprehensible that in 1970 we are still debating the relationship
of carcinoma *in-situ* to invasive cancer', and M.J. Jordan noted: '[I]t can
be stated unequivocally that the Papanicolaou smear has done more
to eradicate invasive cancer of the cervix and lower the death rate from
cancer in women than in any other scientific contribution to date.' None
of the distinguished contributors offered any support to Green, although
one generously suggested his 'iconoclastic' views might be considered 'not
proved'.[22]

In the early 1960s, well before Green had gained approval for his study,
Boyes, Fidler and Lock in Vancouver published evidence suggesting that
organised cervical screening in British Columbia, and treatment of smear-
detected cancer-precursor lesions such as CIS, led to a decreased incidence
of cervical cancer.[23] Green believed that screening in New Zealand had

not had any effect on cervical cancer incidence.[24] Boyes told me that Green invited himself to Vancouver in 1963, where he presented his data. According to Boyes, Green claimed that

> *Professor Richard Doll had assured him [Green] the studies [Canadian and New Zealand] were comparable. I lunched with Professor Doll two months later and he [said he] had never heard of Green. I sent Professor Doll copies of the two papers and he wrote [to] me ... there was no comparison between the two studies, i.e., one population-based and large, and one hospital-based and small. Later that year, Dr Green made the same statement at a gynaecological meeting and Dr H K F Fidler had a copy of my letter from Professor Doll. He read this letter to the audience and Dr Green laughed. 'It was worth a try,' he said.*

During another conversation with Green, Boyes was left with the impression that Green had been an All Black! Green spent some time in Boyes' unit and lectured to staff, but did not endear himself to them because of the 'directness' of his criticism of Boyes, particularly on his 'home ground'. Boyes described him as 'arrogant, bombastic, and with unshakeable views'.[25]

Green was also drawn to Professor Hugh McLaren's unit in Birmingham because McLaren was the leading British advocate of cervical screening. Physically the two men had much in common, but they held diametrically opposed views on the nature of CIS and the potential benefits of screening. McLaren could not understand why Green 'persisted in burying his head in the sand in the light of the evidence in the 1960s and 1970s and the weight of world opinion'.[26] McLaren regarded Green as stubborn and unprepared to evaluate the scientific evidence or the views of his peers. Both Joe Jordan and John Murphy recall 'violent confrontation and disagreement' with McLaren during Green's presentations in Birmingham.[27] Professor Denis Hawkins, who had earlier worked with Bonham at University College Hospital, recalled Green 'facing heavy criticism for his highly unethical and dangerous study' when he lectured at the Royal Postgraduate Medical School at Hammersmith Hospital.[28]

None of these international criticisms surfaced in Auckland – McIndoe was acquainted with them only when he travelled. At home, he studied Green's publications in minute detail and continued to document the outcome in all women diagnosed with CIS in the hospital. In 1973 McIndoe withdrew his colposcopy services from Green's study, although he continued to monitor the outcome of the women. The visiting members of the senior medical staff continued to treat their patients, while Green continued only to observe his.

Michael Churchouse has vivid memories of teaching the basics of cytology to sixth-year medical students, who would then attend Green's lecture on cervical cancer. Returning to Churchouse's office, they would 'poke their heads in the door and say gleefully, "Well, Michael, you may as well pack up and go home – Herb Green has just told us cytology screening is a total waste of time."' Churchouse also recalled Green commenting to him at a hospital Christmas party, 'You know, Michael, when you die nobody will know you are gone, but when I die I will be famous for being the only specialist who held out for the theory that carcinoma *in-situ* and invasive cancer of the cervix are two separate entities with different aetiologies.'[29]

Green's scepticism about cervical screening and the 'premalignant' nature of CIS had a significant adverse influence on the development of cytology screening in New Zealand during the 1960s, 1970s and into the 1980s. Green argued his case in the international scientific literature and also vigorously promoted his 'atypical viewpoint' in the New Zealand press. In a 1970 *New Zealand Herald* article titled 'Cancer smear test overrated', Green was quoted as saying: 'A positive cervical smear test showing "*in-situ*" or dormant-type cancer in a woman is no more likely to develop into "invasive" or malignant cancer of the cervix than in any other woman of the same age in the population.' He also stated that 'a similar type of microscopic appearance to adult *in-situ* cancer ... can be demonstrated in the cervix of [stillborn] infants'. In 1972 the *Herald* quoted Green as saying: 'There is no positive evidence ... cervical smears are a reliable test for cancer.' In an *Auckland Star* newspaper article headlined 'Doubts about the wisdom of mass cancer screening', Green reasserted his contention that '*in-situ* cancer is not a forerunner of invasive cancer'. The article went on to note: 'Professor Green's colleagues at NWH do not necessarily agree with his findings.'[30]

McIndoe regarded Green's public criticism of cytology as 'implied questioning of the credibility and integrity of Dr Williams and me', and set out his detailed response to the criticisms in a memorandum to the medical superintendent: 'It is not reasonable to expect members of the public to appreciate there is a difference between "mass screening" and "cytology as a diagnostic discipline".'[31] Both McIndoe and Dr Stephen Williams, then charge cytopathologist at NWH, challenged Green's views in the correspondence columns of the *New Zealand Medical Journal* in 1972.[32] Dr Ed Giesen, a Wellington gynaecologist, provided support for the two men: 'The time has come for some counter to be made to statements emanating from Auckland [i.e. Green] from time to time to the effect that cervical cytology is of little value.' Giesen's letter provoked a response from Green supporting the case for 'diagnostic' cytology in invasive cervical cancer while questioning 'the wholesale and very expensive screening of asymptomatic populations with the avowed aim of abolishing death from cervical cancer'. Giesen retorted: 'Professor Green is entitled to his opinion, but it must be realised the vast majority of world authorities do not share it.'[33]

In 1972 Dr Ian Ronayne, a supportive colleague of McIndoe, tabled a letter on the agenda of the NWH Senior Medical Staff Committee: 'In view of the recent criticisms in the press on the value of cytology, I feel this matter should be discussed ...' But the recorded minutes stated only: 'The question of possible harm arising from recent articles in the lay press was discussed.'[34] The brevity of the minutes suggests members of the committee were not open to frank discussion of the local criticisms by Green.

Several times Green rebuked McIndoe privately – both in Ward 9 and in Green's office – for comments he had made. On one of these occasions Liggins came into the room and made a comment to the effect, 'Are you two still at it?' In 1976, when NWH radiologist Dr John Stewart visited senior academic and journal editor Professor Dick Mattingly in his gynaecological cancer department in Milwaukee, the latter told him to tell Green to stop his experiment. Stewart, however, never confronted Green: 'It would have been of no use.'[35]

The public and the profession were understandably confused. The Cancer Society was actively promoting mass cervical screening while a senior university professor was publicly stating that such screening was a waste of time and money.

In 1971 Williams wrote to cytopathologist Dr George Wied in Chicago about Green's 'almost obsessional' view regarding CIS:

It is unfortunate ... and there is no doubt ... his emphatically expressed attitude, coming as it does from an influential department, has brought confusion to the local scene.

I believe ... he is sincere, although perhaps bigoted, on this subject. He bases his conclusions on the statistical interpretations and extrapolations of a smallish series of cases, the composition of which has been questioned. It appears that in a number of cases where invasion has clearly followed the original in-situ *diagnosis, he has reviewed the histology himself (although he is not a trained histopathologist) and has removed them from his series on the grounds ... they were invasive carcinomas from the outset.*

There is no doubt ... he has created a good deal of uncertainty amongst the general practitioners and medical students. Altogether it is an embarrassing and awkward development, and one which does not appear to be susceptible to reasoned argument and discussion.[36]

In 1978 Professor Alan Clarke, from the Department of Surgery at the Otago Medical School, commented on a lay article by Green and challenged his 'iconoclastic views', pointing out that 'readers might be mistaken if they saw the article as an objective scientific review simply because it had been written by an academic'.[37] It is noteworthy that, with the exception of Clarke, the only public criticisms of Green in New Zealand at that time were made by non-academics.

But Green refused to budge. As late as 1980, in the words of Dr Mee Ling Yeong, then a young pathologist, 'Ignoring the prevailing teaching, he was almost messianic in his eagerness to spread his gospel, particularly to sceptics [of his position].' She was 'one such sceptic, although a timid one'. She had been taught that CIS preceded invasive cancer 'when the precursor lesion acquired the ability to invade the basement membrane and become a cancer':

Green and I often stopped in the laboratory or corridors of the hospital to discuss the relationship between the two lesions, but it was difficult for a not-yet-qualified 5'2" pathologist to argue her case against the authority of a towering professor with a big booming voice and an unwavering conviction.

One day Professor Green invited me to look down a microscope in his room where he had placed a sample of cervix that contained carcinoma in-situ *on the surface and an invasive cancer in the deeper tissues. There did not appear to be a physical connection between the two lesions in the tissue sample, and this, said Green triumphantly, was surely proof that the two were separate and different diseases. It was no use my trying to explain to the professor that we were looking at a two-dimensional image of a three-dimensional structure. If the technician preparing the slide were to keep cutting into the tissue piece, we would soon see the carcinoma* in-situ *stream into, and connect with, the invasive cancer. Professor Green was in denial.*[38]

In a 1981 paper titled 'Cervical cancer in New Zealand: A failure of cytology?' Green continued to cast doubt on the 'progression model' and the value of cytology screening in the control of cervical cancer.[39] Graeme Duncan, a gynaecologist, was an enthusiastic supporter of cervical cytology, introducing screening to inpatients in Wellington Hospital, teaching colposcopy and founding the New Zealand Colposcopy Society. He also challenged Green's opinion on the relationship between cervical cytology and cervical cancer incidence.[40]

New Zealand obstetricians and gynaecologists generally were not influenced by Green in their own practices, although, as associate professor and deputy head of the Postgraduate School of Obstetrics and Gynaecology, he 'had a significant impact on medical opinion and practice relating to cervical screening'.[41] He occasionally defended his position on the natural history of CIS and screening with complex mathematical models and data analyses, with some of his data described by two experts as 'almost uninterpretable'.[42]

McIndoe meanwhile continued to document his increasing concerns about the welfare of the women in Green's experiment in his private notes. On 14 July 1971, for example, he wrote:

The scene in Ward 9 Theatre Room today on the appearance of Mrs T who has been under observation since 24-10-68 seems to have stimulated Mr Harbutt alarmingly.

To me we are seeing what will be an increasingly common phenomenon over the next few months as time runs on and patients come up for biopsy who have been inadequately biopsied over the last few years.

The staff must grapple with the present problem and see ... responsibility for the present situation does not shift from where it truly lies at the moment.[43]

Days later Harbutt gave McIndoe a list of 28 women he wished to 'review' who had originally presented with smear abnormalities – some later developed cancer. There is no record of the outcome of Harbutt's request.[44]

* * *

So what was it like for the hundreds of women who attended Green's clinic? Those who thought Green was doing good, saving his patients from 'unnecessary surgery', were ignoring the fact that his approach involved multiple mutilating cervical biopsies aimed at excluding cancer. These resulted in significant scarring, infertility and inability to obtain optimal cervical smears, and sometimes translated an otherwise overt cancer to a more serious covert lesion.

Many women travelled long distances by train or bus from the poorer parts of Auckland, often with small children in tow; few had cars. Sometimes husbands had to take time off from work to transport their wives or care for children. Patients attended the clinic every three to six months, or at least annually: some attended over a period of 20 years. Ironically, many women interpreted the frequent and often inconvenient hospital visits as evidence of the ever-watchful eye of a caring doctor when, in fact, the object of their visit was to enable that doctor to exclude the presence of developing cancer.

After queuing to confirm their attendance, the women were directed to sit in the long, narrow, Clinic 1 corridor. Often after a lengthy wait they were directed to a tiny cubicle, told to strip and put on a white gown; they then had to wait until a couch was available. When their turn came they were told to lie on an examination couch and were covered with a cream sheet. The green curtains at the end of the couch were then flung back and Green or a resident medical officer would appear, often accompanied by medical students. Some women, grateful for the professor's care, would bring him small gifts of home-grown produce, jams, eggs or pickles. It was soon time for 'Knees up, knees apart', cold speculum, smear and then 'We will see you again in six months'. Some women were told they would be directed to McIndoe for a colposcopy, and some were informed they would be admitted for another biopsy, but many were never contacted with their smear results – normal or abnormal, later learning the outcome from their family doctor or on their next visit to the clinic – maybe.

* * *

The fourth important person now enters the story.

Dr Malcolm McLean, or Jock as he was known, was appointed charge pathologist at NWH in 1961. A tall, well-built man with a florid complexion and a military bearing, he wore country-style check shirts with ties, tweed jackets with patches on the elbows, and brogues. He was 'too big' for his green Scimitar sports car. On first meeting he appeared reserved, a characteristic enhanced by his tendency to blink involuntarily when with strangers or when under stress. In many respects he epitomised the professional pathologist working in a basement laboratory office, spending his day peering through a microscope.

Over two decades McLean was served well by two secretaries, Jane Cumming and Gloria McGuire, who described him as unusual, complex, unpretentious – a man who played up to and fulfilled everyone's expectations about his eccentricity. His pet phrase was: 'Scratch my surface and you will find the real me underneath.' He enjoyed fraternising with his laboratory staff and flirting with women, but regarded the establishment as 'stuffed shirts'. His secretaries described him as being 'very particular with his work', also noting that they were sent out of his office if there was an issue of confidentiality. He often likened colleagues on the medical staff who privately supported his and McIndoe's stand against Green to 'penguins on an ice floe – they push one in first and if he doesn't get eaten by the killer whales they all jump in'. From 1975 he became, in his own words, 'obsessed with Green's experiment'.[45]

In Bryan Trenwith's view, 'Jock's main interest was in the cone biopsy slides which arrived on his desk in vast numbers from the histology section of the laboratory [and] were reviewed at regular intervals by Prof Herb Green and his team.'

Fierce arguments between Jock and Herb would occur. Herb would disagree with Jock when his histology report had cast doubt on Herb's theory that carcinoma in-situ *was a separate disease entity and did not progress to invasive cancer of the cervix. These meetings were full of tension; Herb would arrive pale-faced – a tall, imposing man, often with the hint of a small froth of saliva at the corner of his mouth ... he was a most formidable proponent of his point of view. He held forth about his 'Woman' – he never used the plural of the word! Meanwhile Jock vigorously defended the reports he had made on his 'Ladies'.*

After one of these sessions, Green noticed me in the laboratory and remembered that I had been at National Women's as a student. He asked me about my experience in histology and I told him it was not great. Then he asked me if I would report on the slides from his patients who had had biopsies of the cervix; I gathered the aim was to bypass Jock and avoid what Herb considered to be his erroneous interpretations. I was taken aback by this suggestion and declined to take part.[46]

This was a remarkable exchange. Green, who would later claim to possess the skills of a specialist gynaecological pathologist, was considering bypassing McLean and entering into collaboration with a first-year pathology registrar.

McLean's spacious office, situated at the laboratory entrance, over-looked a grassed area opposite Ward 9, the ward reserved for Green's cancer patients. The office had a circumferential bench adjacent to the wall with a large central table almost filling the room. The only seating was two elevated stools adjacent to the microscope – one for McLean and the other for colleagues or student doctors who came to discuss the pathology of cases of particular interest. A screen on one wall allowed teaching images to be projected from a modified microscope sitting on the central table.

Every inch of McLean's desk was covered with piles of medical journals, scientific papers – many of which had been photocopied for him by McIndoe, cardboard boxes filled with glass slides from current patients, and referral slides from other New Zealand pathologists requesting a second opinion. The piles of paper extended from his laboratory office to cover a full-sized billiard table in the basement of his Epsom home.

He was appointed as foundation clinical teacher in pathology when the Auckland Medical School was established in 1969. An excellent and much-respected teacher, McLean was remembered for the detailed preparation of his lectures and deft use of up to three slide projectors simultaneously.[47] His well-ordered mind and strong, clear voice sent unambiguous messages even with complex material. He made the addition of the suffix '-oid' to words – an arrangement of cells resembling a cartwheel would become 'cartwheel-oid' – his particular speciality. A continual stream of laboratory technicians, registrars-in-training and colleagues created constant interruptions. Unfortunately McLean's later years were marred by health problems.

McLean came from a working-class family and, like McIndoe, attended Auckland Grammar School. This was followed by army service. After demobilisation he obtained a Returned Serviceman's Bursary enabling him to attend Otago Medical School. He graduated in 1949 and did a four-year residency at Auckland Hospital during which time he married Ailsa, a science graduate and his perfect foil. He then went to Greymouth Hospital on the West Coast, a 'special area' hospital, as its first pathologist. During this time he completed a Doctor of Medicine degree.

The earliest biological pregnancy tests involved injecting a woman's urine into a female rabbit, and then a few days later killing it and examining its ovaries. These would alter if a hormone secreted only by pregnant women was present. Later, frogs were used, because they did not need to be killed. Since McLean did not like killing rabbits, as had happened at Auckland Hospital, he elected to use the frog test. He and Ailsa failed to catch any frogs in Greymouth's wetlands, so advertised in the *Grey River Argus* for the amphibians at one shilling each. The hospital was inundated with hundreds of frogs and dozens of little boys all demanding their shillings.[48]

McLean's time at Grey Hospital provided him with additional funds for two years of postgraduate pathology study in London. Initially he worked in Professor John Dacie's haematology service at the Royal Postgraduate Medical School at Hammersmith Hospital, then in Sir Roy Cameron's research laboratory at University College Hospital. McLean was a foundation member of the Royal College of Pathologists, a Fellow of the Royal College of Pathologists of Australia and a member of the International College of Pathologists.

He returned to Hutt Hospital as a general pathologist before joining NWH as a specialist gynaecological pathologist in 1961. Like McIndoe, he was one of the few people to witness directly the outcomes in women involved in Green's study. Anxious to establish more open dialogue on the problem, he wrote to the medical superintendent in 1971, suggesting the establishment of a 'tumour panel' 'of interested members of the senior [medical] staff'. He set out his vision in a memorandum:

Aims to be as follows:

- *to allow the fullest possible use of individual expertise and experience for the diagnosis and management of patients with tumours, particularly rarities and difficult cases.*
- *to keep appropriate records and to inform other members of the staff of up-to-date trends, findings and results in this field.*
- *to consider the setting up of a National Gynaecological Tumour registry.*

As he pointed out, 'Optimum tumour management is a complex problem and patients have every right to expect the best the hospital can provide. It is beyond the ability of any one individual these days to be fully versed in all its aspects.' He was also aware that, although there was 'room for study and investigation with the aim of improving diagnosis and management', caution was needed 'where patient interests are at stake ... Controversial and difficult cases need to be discussed openly.'[49] McLean's suggestion led to the establishment of New Zealand's first multidisciplinary gynaecological Tumour Panel.

In many ways McIndoe and McLean had strikingly different personalities, yet they shared strong professional integrity and a warm humanity for their patients. And both had one advantage: they spent much of their professional lives looking at cancer cells through a microscope. With the exception of Green and his immediate staff, who were examining patients in a clinic, no one else was coming face to face with cancer cells on a daily basis.

McLean introduced the term 'creeping kiss' to describe the progressive extension, over time, of untreated CIS lesions 'creeping' over larger areas of skin, sometimes extending from the cervix to cover the vagina, vulva, urethra and perianal skin. Treatment became progressively more difficult with an increasing risk of invasive cancer.

While the women in Green's study were unaware of the concerns McIndoe and McLean had for them, Ailsa McLean saw the stress the experiment was causing her husband. McLean was in a good position to monitor Green's study, observing as he was at microscopic level the persistence of CIS or the progression to invasive cancer in some patients. Ailsa McLean elected to bypass the NWH authorities and go directly to medical superintendent-in-chief Dr Wilton Henley with her concerns. She later recalled her agitation as she poured out her worries. Henley tried to calm her, promising he would look into the matter, but there is no evidence that any action resulted.[50] Henley was the first – but not the last – medical superintendent-in-chief who failed to respond to concerns raised about Green's experiment.

CHAPTER 5

WHITEWASH

Cancer is life, albeit in a disorganised form, and attempts to find a solution to the problem of cancer must be regarded as attempts to find a solution to the problem of life itself. The problem is almost a metaphysical one.

HERBERT GREEN, 1974

WHEN I ARRIVED at NWH in 1973 there was considerable discussion about and media interest in a new and controversial form of cancer treatment being performed by Milan Brych in the radiotherapy department at Auckland Hospital. Brych received support from the highest levels of the medical profession, including the Director General of Health, Dr John Hiddlestone, and the medical superintendent-in-chief, Dr Fred Moody. Brych's treatment involved intermittent 'bolus' chemotherapy and a secret form of 'immunotherapy'.

As tutor specialist I was asked to organise a 'Clinical Problems' meeting to 'address the staff on the subject of the "immunotherapy" treatment of cancer' with special reference to that being performed on NWH patients at Auckland Hospital.[1] This was not the usual clinical meeting: the lecture theatre was packed; there was tension and a sense of anticipation in the air. At the time there were differing opinions among medical staff of both Brych and his controversial treatments. Dr Pat Dunn, the gynaecologist at NWH who had performed earlier surgery on the patient Brych was to present to the meeting, was most impressed by the outcome of the therapy and had written a supportive letter to Brych, and subsequently to the newspapers.[2]

On 19 April 1973 Dr Ross Burton, head of the radiotherapy department, and Brych addressed 38 senior medical staff and many resident medical officers from NWH and other Auckland hospitals. In his opening remarks Burton said he had given Hiddlestone and Moody an undertaking not to reveal the secret nature of Brych's 'immunotherapy' treatment and added he did not want Brych to be pilloried at the meeting.[3] Brych and Burton beamed when Dunn's patient described the dramatic disappearance, following the chemo/immunotherapy, of a large secondary tumour in her neck from a previously treated uterine sarcoma. (It was subsequently revealed that the resolution of the tumour was the result of chemotherapy alone.) There was considerable scepticism among the audience, and many 'direct and searching questions'. When Brych explained that he actively 'immunised' patients by injecting a tumour-specific antigen, Mont Liggins accused him, to his face, of being a charlatan. Later Burton described the meeting as a vulgar 'brawl' and said 'there was a claque following us around offering destructive criticism'.[4]

Concern regarding Brych's qualifications and controversial therapy led to a ministerial inquiry initiated by Sir Harcourt Caughey, chairman of the Auckland Hospital Board.[5] It became evident that Brych's secret study was experimental and had never been referred to the Auckland Hospital Ethics Committee. Brych was indeed a charlatan. He had been in prison for robbery with violence during the seven years he claimed to be receiving his medical training; his 'immunotherapy' claims were fraudulent. Professor Douglas Wright, from Melbourne, who chaired the eventual public inquiry into Brych's bogus therapy, visited NWH and directed the Hospital Board 'to leave the strong points of excellence, such as the obstetric and gynaecological cancer care, treatment and research to develop where it is well advanced'. Clearly, those advising on cancer research at NWH had made a strong impression on Wright.[6] Professors John Scott, John Buchanan and Dr Gordon Nicholson, who raised the alarm, investigated and established the case against Brych, all encountered considerable difficulty in obtaining support from senior medical staff and administrators. In the university medical faculty, Buchanan received the most support from Bonham and Green.[7]

* * *

My first professional discussion with Green occurred over lunch in the medical staff dining room early in 1973. He had probably read my CV and, having ascertained that I was trained in both surgery and obstetrics and gynaecology, he may have sensed that I was a surgically oriented doctor with an interest in cancer. I was vaguely aware of his controversial views on the nature of CIS, but ignorant of the growing concerns among some of his colleagues about his experiment. As a young specialist I had many areas of interest; CIS and its management was only one of them. Dealing with obstetric and gynaecological emergencies was to be my priority for the next three years.

Following pleasantries I was surprised how soon Green broached the subject of CIS of the cervix. This was obviously his passion and he was no doubt anxious to establish whether this newcomer might be a potential ally. I briefly presented the conventional view that CIS was a precancer and should be treated, and intimated that if a colposcopy service was available it should be used together with a biopsy examination to confirm the diagnosis before treatment. Green listened to my views without interruption, then proceeded to make stringent criticisms of conventional teaching and the limitations of cytology, pathology and epidemiology, providing me with a stream of confusing data and statistics, including evidence from his own research.

Who was I to challenge these views? I was sitting with a man who claimed a lifetime of experience of caring for women with CIS – indeed, an authority on the subject, albeit one with an unconventional viewpoint. This man deserved my respect and I could learn from him. On the other hand I was somewhat intimidated and conscious of my youth and inexperience. Despite these reservations, and notwithstanding his gruff manner, I felt that Green made me welcome in my new hospital. A few months later he invited Barbara and me to a party at his Epsom home to meet Harvey Carey, the previous postgraduate professor, who was visiting Auckland.

At the Cartwright Inquiry Professor Colin Mantell would emphasise the exemplary care received by women in Green's ward. There was no hospice care in those days. Women with terminal cancer were frequently readmitted back into the ward where they had previously received their cancer treatment.

Ward 9 was a single-room ward with mixed patronage. There were women who were undergoing treatment for cervical cancer, or dying from it. Sister Isobel Fisher remembered nursing 13 women who died of the disease during a two-week period. Families of women receiving radium treatment were not allowed to visit the patients in their rooms because of the radiation risk; instead they stood outside in all weathers, waving through the windows. Side-rooms in the ward were reserved for women with septic gynaecological conditions. On occasion Liggins, an innovative surgeon, used these beds for his male patients undergoing sex-change operations. Sister Fisher objected to the presence in her ward of these men with 'large shoulders, wearing flimsy nighties'.[8]

Terminal care was largely based on personal warmth, good nursing and liberal dosing with a drug mixture known as a Brompton's cocktail. In pharmacist Ray Laurie's words, the pharmacy on the Cornwall Hospital site 'had a very good relationship with Professor Green – no doubt due to the close proximity of the professorial unit to the pharmacy. Our staff liked Professor Green very much as during his visits to the pharmacy he impressed with the care and interest he showed for his patients.'

Professor Green used to get annoyed that the local drug addicts had access to heroin, while his patients were denied this medicine due to an international agreement not to import the drug. Heroin was credited with producing greater euphoria for patients in severe pain. Pain appeared to lessen addiction which was not a problem anyway, while complications such as nausea and constipation were lessened. 'Professor Green's Mixture', which was frequently charted, consisted of heroin – diamorphine HCl (later morphine sulphate) 10 mg, cocaine HCl 10 mg, and chlorpromazine HCl 25 mg in either 5 or 10 ml largactil. The 'Brompton Mixture', which was essentially the same formula, possibly with more alcohol of the patient's liking, made the dying patient more sociable in their last days.[9]

Green approached Glyn Richards, a young anaesthetist with skills in modern pain management, and told him how regretful he was that heroin (diamorphine) was no longer available. Richards, who was 'always very impressed by the standard of medical nursing care in [Green's] unit', recalled one patient in particular.

One young woman, who was receiving treatment for advanced cervical cancer, had just completed a Bachelor of Arts degree and should at that time have been looking forward to going to her capping ceremony. Her illness clearly prevented it. I was surprised to be approached by Prof Green who told me he wanted to arrange a capping ceremony for her on the ward, and could I, along with others, attend in suitable academic dress. I was fortunate to be able to borrow my university gown and faculty cape from an older colleague, who had attended the same North of England University. We assembled on the day and made a colourful procession of faculty and graduate gowns and capes, down the corridor to the young lady's bedside. She was duly capped and presented with her degree. The ceremony was suitably 'capped off' with tea and cakes.[10]

* * *

On meeting McIndoe I was immediately drawn to his warm, friendly manner and his enthusiasm for his field of interest. At first we did not discuss his concerns relating to Green's experiment; I was keen to become involved in colposcopy and McIndoe recognised a kindred spirit. Initially I shared a clinic, observing and learning from him. Later I worked in a separate clinic alongside him. After a short time he broached the topic of Green's research and became excited as he shared his description of the experiment and his concerns – our conversations continued until his death 13 years later.

Unlike my initial encounters with McIndoe, my early contacts with McLean were formal – a clinician seeking advice from a colleague on the pathology of a specimen from a patient I had operated upon, or discussion of cases to be presented at a forthcoming Tumour Panel. Later I began to appreciate that the close professional relationship between McIndoe and McLean was based, not only on their respective professional responsibilities, but also on their concern for the women in Green's study. McIndoe had received some formal pathology training and so was keen to share McLean's microscope and discuss the relationship between his observations of the smear test and the biopsy (histology) of the tissue – a multidisciplinary approach.

In September 1973, nine months after my arrival at NWH, McIndoe invited me to join him and Green at a special colposcopy clinic on the occasion of the visit of Professor Per Kolstad, Head of Gynaecological Cancer at the Norwegian Radium Hospital in Oslo and one of only a handful of internationally recognised colposcopists. I felt privileged to be invited. Kolstad was a somewhat dour, balding man of above average build, with penetrating grey eyes. McIndoe, who had befriended Kolstad at international colposcopy meetings, had invited him to New Zealand specifically to acquaint him with the problems arising from Green's study. Kolstad had earlier written:

> *Evidence at hand, both from retrospective and prospective studies and from population screening projects indicate that no more than 30% of women to whom the histologic diagnosis of carcinoma* in-situ *is assigned would ever develop invasive cancer, even if left untreated. ... [and] it is not justified to allow a patient to go without treatment when a diagnosis of carcinoma* in-situ *has been made.*[11]

This was the only occasion I witnessed Green and McIndoe working together in a clinical setting. Although relations between the two men had largely broken down by this time, there was no obvious tension: they acted in the civil, professional manner expected when consulting with patients in the presence of an international authority.

Kolstad began by demonstrating the technique of colposcopy on four uncontentious cases – women presenting with smear abnormalities and requiring treatment. Green also allowed McIndoe to bring two women 'on follow-up with continuing cervical and vaginal lesions' (CIS) for Kolstad's opinion.[12] At the end of the colposcopy clinic a further six of Green's cases with continuing smear abnormalities were discussed. Kolstad found it difficult, as a visitor in a host hospital, to control his incredulity at the way these latter women had been neglected. Nonetheless, he made it abundantly clear to McIndoe and Green that these women should be treated, even at this late stage. As he pointed out to McIndoe and me later, treatment at the outset would have been relatively straightforward; now it was associated with significant risks.[13]

Later McIndoe confirmed in a letter to the medical superintendent, Algar Warren, that Kolstad had described Green as 'experimenting with patients'. Kolstad also told McIndoe he was free to cite 'my opinions about carcinoma *in-situ* treatment methods, and the responsibility of the doctors handling the cases'. On his return home Kolstad wrote to McIndoe: 'I am sorry to [learn] about your trouble at the hospital … and [I am] critical of what is happening …'[14] McIndoe would have welcomed some more concrete advice on how to deal with the problem. Kolstad also discussed his concerns about Green's study with Dr Margaret Davy, a young Australian gynaecologist then working at his unit in Oslo. She recalled later that Kolstad's first concern was always for the welfare of patients.[15]

Immediately after Kolstad's visit, McIndoe, followed shortly by McLean, wrote further memoranda to Warren, setting out in unambiguous terms their concerns relating to Green's failure to manage adequately women with CIS. McIndoe's letter of 10 October 1973 stated:

> I have not been entirely happy, for a number of years, with the management of many patients who have had abnormal cytology and colposcopy findings … I expressed my disagreement with this policy at the Senior Medical Staff meeting [20 June 1966]. For a time following this meeting I began to wonder whether I had been unnecessarily

concerned. However the subsequent clinical course of a number of patients having varying forms of conservative care leads me to believe that a reappraisal of policy towards management of patients with abnormal cytology and colposcopy findings is called for.

He attached a list of the names of seven women who had developed cancer under Green's policy of observation. There was also a document summarising the erratic phases of Green's management of women with CIS, Green's personal criticisms of McIndoe, and his criticisms of cytology. Appended to this 12-page memorandum were 55 pages of supporting documents, including a number of scientific papers.[16]

To this point McIndoe had maintained the usual professional courtesies with Green, politely addressing his concerns verbally and in writing, followed by informal discussion with senior colleagues. None of this had resulted in any reappraisal of the 1966 experiment. Now, with the added impetus of Kolstad's forthright rejection of Green's experiment, in McIndoe's judgement it was time for Warren to investigate.

McLean's memorandum to the medical superintendent followed eight days later. The thrust of his letter was that observation of women with evidence of continuing abnormalities, who had originally had only small diagnostic biopsies, led to delays in the diagnosis of cancer. McLean went on to restate the widely recognised observation: 'The majority of cases of early [cervical] carcinoma are associated with carcinoma *in-situ.*' He appended a list of the names of 13 women with inadequate biopsies who had been subjected to delays before the diagnosis of cancer.[17]

Warren forwarded McIndoe's and McLean's memoranda to Green through his head of department, Bonham. Green began his response to Warren by saying, 'I am prepared to comment on this despite my astonishment at the manner in which [the] two staff members have chosen to approach this matter.' He went on to address the subjective opinions of pathologists and to state that in his study there was 'a calculated risk that invasive cancer may be overlooked'.[18] Green had not suggested any such risk when he submitted the proposal for his study in 1966. He proceeded to describe his personal experience in the histology of 1050 cases of cervical cancer, stating boldly: 'I am intimately concerned with the history and clinical findings in many patients, their histological sections, their treatment, and their follow-up – so … I am in a better position to say what or might not happen to a given patient.'[19] Green was the captain of this ship; McIndoe and McLean were merely crew.

McIndoe quickly responded in a letter to Warren:

It was not possible to approach this matter in any other way because of the personality and belligerent response of Associate Professor Green to comment and criticism.

It was quite incorrect to state ... I have never made plain my feelings ... [but] he not only will not, but does not, listen to any comment which does not suit him. I have endeavoured by all means possible in a mature and dignified manner to make my feelings plain and so note down specific instances of my attempts.[20]

Bonham, who had been privy to this correspondence, immediately wrote a 'confidential document' of uncertain distribution titled, 'Cancer management at National Women's Hospital'.[21] In the section on CIS of the cervix he wrote that its relationship 'to the true invasive cancer of the cervix remains an enigma'. Did Bonham really believe that or was he simply providing dutiful support for Green?

Unlike Green, who brazened out the controversies surrounding him, McIndoe took it all to heart. He wrestled with his conscience over many issues, particularly anguishing over the fate of women in Green's care. On more than one occasion he took stress leave to distance himself from Green and the increasingly concerning sequelae of the experiment.

McLean wisely allowed six months for tempers to 'cool' and in order to give the matter 'deep consideration'. Where Green, alone, determined the diagnosis and management the patient was to receive, McLean, the pathologist, took the perspective of the patient. His reply of 18 October 1973 read:

I reaffirm my concern over his [Green's] extremely conservative approach to the diagnosis and management of cases purported to be carcinoma in-situ of the cervix.

When patients are admitted to a public hospital they put themselves in the hands of the medical staff with explicit understanding they will be provided with at least adequate, and preferably optimal, treatment for their complaint. Clinical studies and trials to establish optimal management are at times necessary. However, when in the course of a trial it becomes apparent patients are at risk, there must be a reappraisal

of the trial. Despite what Professor Green may say, the consensus of
opinion at present is that any delay in the diagnosis and treatment of
invasive carcinoma puts the patient at an increased risk.[22]

In response Green wrote, 'Dr McLean is entitled to his opinion, even on clinical matters if he so chooses (and he has so chosen), but similarly I must be allowed my opinion on histological matters. Dr McLean hardly ever sees the patients before treatment, and never in their follow-up care.'[23]

McIndoe's daughter, Mary Whaley, remembered clearly her father's anxiety regarding his subsequent visit, with McLean and Warren, to Dr Fred Moody, the medical superintendent-in-chief, to express his concerns about Green's experiment. Moody declined to become involved and referred the matter back to the Hospital Medical Committee for investigation, observing that 'there appears to be evidence to suggest there is misrepresentation of histological and clinical findings – possibly to the detriment of patients'.[24] Moody was the second superintendent-in-chief who chose not to become involved.

* * *

Although the reports of McIndoe, McLean and Green were tabled at the Hospital Medical Committee and Senior Medical Staff Committee meetings, no one really seemed to know what to do with them. Finally, 19 months after McIndoe's first memorandum to the superintendent, a subcommittee comprising two senior members of the visiting staff, Alastair Macfarlane and Bernard Kyle, and Associate Professor Richard Seddon, was invited 'to look at the case notes of certain specified cases to assess whether they were managed in accordance with the accepted hospital practice at this time'.

Kyle responded: 'As I believe medical progress throughout the centuries has been impeded by people making decisions about subjects on which they know nothing, I beg to decline the opportunity to serve on the Committee in question.' After he was again invited to join the committee, he replied: 'Furthermore I feel it is most inappropriate … that this matter should be adjudicated upon by members of this hospital staff because of the personalities and the fact that local staff have had a long time in which to prejudge the issue.' Despite concerns that 'it may be uneconomic of time and money', he thought 'this problem would be better assessed by a Gynaecologist, Pathologist and Oncologist from some other institution'.[25]

A suggestion by Kyle and Ronayne that John Monaghan from Newcastle, England, be invited to review the cases was not accepted. Kyle's statements provided very clear guidance to Warren and the Hospital Medical Committee, but they did not heed it. Dr Bruce Faris, another senior member of the visiting staff, replaced Kyle on the committee. Macfarlane and Faris were both longstanding professional colleagues and friends of Green; Seddon had been a student of Green and was now a colleague in the academic department. Soon after, Seddon moved to a new professorial chair in Wellington. The committee did not seek independent expert advice.

Twenty-nine cases of concern were referred to the subcommittee for review. The chairman, Alastair Macfarlane, excluded 15 without recording a reason for doing so, and another case was excluded because the woman had entered the study before it officially began in 1966. The subcommittee of three examined the records of the remaining 13 cases, all of whom had developed invasive cancer (one had already died). Even though the subcommittee developed its own terms of reference, it stated that 'it is not within the terms of reference of the committee to comment on the outcome of the clinical trial to which the agreed policy applies'. Note the description of Green's study as a 'trial'.

In its report of 18 September 1975 the subcommittee considered it 'regrettable that differences of professional opinion held by senior staff members have been allowed to result in conflicts which have had to come to arbitration' and was of the 'firm opinion … that all staff members involved in the implementation of the policy concerned with the conservative management of carcinoma-in-situ of the cervix have acted with personal and professional integrity'. It believed that 'the effective continuation of this trial' depended on the staff concerned 'subjugating personality differences in the interests of scientific enquiry'. The initial policy should be 'clarified in accordance with the following recommendations: a) Define whose concern for the safety of the patient is to be acted upon …'[26]

What remarkable statements – 'staff members … have acted with personal and professional integrity', 'subjugating personality differences'. All 13 women in their self-selected review had developed cancer; one had already died. What would it have taken for them to declare the trial a failure?

In my opinion the comments of these men highlight their misplaced loyalty to Green and his 1966 proposal. The subcommittee's report was duly tabled and that was to be the end of the matter. Understandably McIndoe and McLean were upset, though not entirely surprised; it seemed everyone else had anaesthetised their consciences.

The response of Green's colleagues to the in-house working party report was ambivalent. Privately, some referred to it as a 'whitewash' and from that time stopped referring cases to him. On the other hand none had either the foresight or the courage to stop the experiment on the women who remained under Green's care. He blundered on, apparently oblivious to the increasing risks faced by his patients.

As Judge Cartwright was later to observe:

The Hospital Medical Committee and the Working Party should have been thinking of the patients' safety; instead they preferred to follow the time-honoured tradition of confusing etiquette with ethics in attempting to repair the relationships which had deteriorated in the hospital as a result of the 1966 proposal and its consequences for patients.

The instigation of the Working Party's review was the best opportunity the medical staff at National Women's Hospital had to confront the problems which surrounded the 1966 trial and exercise a genuine form of internal peer review. It is apparent right from the beginning, in their self-limiting terms of reference, they chose instead to avoid the real issue. If they had approached their task differently, or if Dr Kyle's recommendations had been acted upon, I do not believe this Inquiry would have been necessary.[27]

Green published his last major paper on the natural history of CIS in the *New Zealand Medical Journal* in 1974, at the time the working party was being set up,[28] but it is not known whether the members read it or were influenced by it. By now McIndoe had become visibly depressed. He drafted a number of responses to the *New Zealand Medical Journal*. In his lengthy and detailed final draft he listed 39 women with progression to cancer, including women with either untreated or inadequately treated CIS and stage 1A cancer. He finished with the comment: 'I am forced to enquire why [Green] has included only part of the material available in the review.' He was again clearly suggesting Green had manipulated the data. He also hinted at a 'forthcoming publication [to be] presented by us in due course'. Sadly the pressure finally got on top of McIndoe; he took stress leave from the hospital and did not submit his critique.[29]

* * *

In 1973 the New Zealand Medical Research Council invited epidemiologist Sir Richard Doll, Regius Professor of Medicine at Oxford, to be the
guest speaker at a seminar in Auckland. Green presented a paper titled
'The progression of so-called preinvasive lesions of the cervix', which
drew on the same flawed data that was published in the *New Zealand
Medical Journal* a year later. The thrust of his address is clear from the
title. Doll remarked that Green's paper

> *was an example of the most useful thing a scientist can do, namely
> the issue of a challenge to generally accepted ideas. Whatever the final
> outcome of his study may be he has succeeded in making us realise
> once again the disastrous power of words [i.e. carcinoma* in-situ*] to
> constrain thought.*[30]

Doll was clearly not familiar with the background to Green's research,
the harm resulting from it or his manipulation of the data. And of course
Green went on to use Doll's remarks later to justify his experiment.
This was the second time in 13 years that Green had falsely cited Doll's
support for his study. In 2002 Doll told me Green 'went wrong in not
keeping a closer eye on the results and not having some colleagues to act
as data monitors'.[31] He little realised that McIndoe and McLean were in
fact performing this task, but that Green was refusing to listen to them.

In 1970 Professor Bruce Baguley, later director of the University of
Auckland Cancer Research Laboratory, was a young research scientist
attending his first international meeting. He was 'approached by an
Australian oncologist who told me how much he admired Herb Green
and his views on cancer'. The following year Green visited the Department
of Cell Biology at Auckland University and gave a talk entitled 'The
cellular theory of cancer'. Baguley recalled:

> *The gist of his talk was that the idea of understanding cancer by
> studying the behaviour of isolated cancer cells was wrong, and the
> only way forward in research was to study cancer as a complete
> tissue. He made the analogy that one 'could not solve the problems of
> Auckland traffic by redesigning the motor car'. Since the main thrust
> of research in the Department of Cell Biology was based on studying
> individual cells, this idea went down like a lead balloon with most of
> my colleagues.*[32]

Baguley met Green afterwards and explained that although he did not agree with everything he said, he was interested in his views. Green responded with an invitation to his office at NWH the following week.

Over a bottle of whisky, the two men had 'a long-ranging discussion, not only about the nature of cancer but also on the Auckland research scene ... As the evening wore on, and perhaps encouraged by the whisky, Herb expressed his deep bitterness about the Auckland Cancer Society's support of a research programme on the development of new anticancer drugs', which he regarded as 'an utter waste of money ... the Cancer Society should be putting its funding exclusively into clinical research.' Although Baguley was part of this programme, headed by Professor Bruce Cain, he detected no 'personal antagonism' from Green and the pair met occasionally over the following years.

Herb Green's main conjecture was that cancer development was governed by a series of interconnected random events, often called a 'stochastic' process. Herb enjoyed talking with me because I had a background in mathematics as well as chemistry and biology, and could therefore speak the same language. Herb's ideas were strongly influenced by other scientists including David Smithers and Philip Burch, and he provided me with various articles and books on this subject. He elaborated his ideas in a commentary published in New Zealand Medical Journal *in [1970] where he suggested the onset of cancer was related to age by a mathematical function and was therefore inevitable. Quoting MacDonald he concluded it was 'biological pre-determinism' rather than the efficacy of treatment that determined the result.[33] This article provides some insight into Herb Green's underlying thinking on cancer; the role of the clinician was to alleviate suffering, but the progression of cancer was independent of treatment.*

It was, Baguley considered, 'inevitable' that Green's ideas would 'conflict with those of Bruce Cain, who thought medicinal chemistry had the potential to cure cancer'. Green, who was 'perhaps emotionally against the latter concept ... even tried to influence the Auckland Cancer Society in order to eliminate their support of Bruce Cain's programme'.[34]

Green's sometimes nihilistic approach to the management of women with cancer is supported by one of his studies suggesting that the duration and type of symptom may be less important in determining the prognosis than generally thought, with the implication that treatment has little influence on the overall outcome.[35] As he wrote in 1974, 'Cancer is life, albeit in a disorganised form, and attempts to find a solution to the problem of cancer must be regarded as attempts to find a solution to the problem of life itself. The problem is almost a metaphysical one.'[36]

In 1975 I attended a presentation by Green titled 'Biological pre-determinism in cervical cancer prognosis' at the centenary meeting of the Otago Medical School. Using data from his follow-up studies of women with invasive cervical cancer, Green argued: 'The results suggest that stage [of a cervical cancer] is predetermined, and delay in diagnosis does not alter the outcome.'[37] The theory of biological predeterminism proposes that the behaviour of a cancer is a consequence of 'randomly occurring biological factors, possibly genetic, which are established in the pre-clinical phase of the disease.'[38] Thus, early diagnosis and treatment do not necessarily confer a survival advantage. This view was clearly contrary to conventional teaching, but consistent with the views Green had expressed to Baguley.

Professor (later Sir) John Stallworthy, the New Zealand-born Professor of Obstetrics and Gynaecology at Oxford University, was awarded an honorary Doctor of Science degree at the meeting. Stallworthy listened to Green's presentation from the back of the steeply tiered lecture theatre, then proceeded to make a vitriolic personal attack on Green and his presentation. None of us in the audience had previously witnessed such a direct attack on a colleague in a major medical meeting – indeed we all felt sorry for Green. Left in no doubt that he was a lone voice, Green nonetheless persisted with his experiment and women continued to suffer in increasing numbers.

The majority of New Zealand's obstetricians and gynaecologists attended the silver jubilee meeting of the Postgraduate School in 1976. Bonham invited Green, McIndoe, McLean and me to contribute to a symposium on cervical cancer.[39] Green himself lectured on 'Assessment of the spectrum of progression theory of cervix lesions', drawing heavily on his 1974 paper, where he stated that only 1.3 per cent of women managed with CIS developed cancer.[40]

Using essentially the same data, McIndoe (with McLean and me) drew quite different conclusions. He reported that 16.6 per cent of women with positive cytology follow-up developed cancer, compared with only 0.7 per cent of women with negative cytology follow-up – data he was shortly to present to the International Federation for Cervical Pathology and Colposcopy in Orlando, Florida. He concluded: 'CIS is clearly a disease of consequence and can have invasive carcinoma potential.'[41] Dr Graeme Duncan from Wellington made a statement supporting McIndoe, McLean and me. The chairman, Dr Bruce Grieve, then invited questions. There were none – no one had the courage to challenge the speakers over the marked differences in cancer rates between Green's and McIndoe's presentations.

I vividly recall the end-of-year party in 1973. The senior medical staff gave a formal black tie, complimentary dinner for junior medical staff in the Victorian splendour of the ivy-covered, male-only Northern Club, as a way of thanking them for their work. Unlike today, when junior medical staff are rostered on duty for set hours, in those days it often meant many days on call, and with much greater responsibilities. Senior medical staff gave formal thank you speeches, while junior wits used the opportunity to gently ridicule the senior staff, which some wives did not appear to appreciate. After the dinner younger doctors either went home or found more exciting entertainment beyond the club; the senior men's wives were invited to an adjacent room for coffee and port while their husbands remained in the dining room, cigars lit, and listened to two senior doctors recite 'The Ballad of Eskimo Nell' and A.P. Herbert's 'Ode to Female Parts'. Male chauvinism was alive and well in this room of older male gynaecologists.

CHAPTER 6

PHOEBE'S STORY

It may become malignant, but I think she is likely to die of something else long before that.

HERBERT GREEN, 1971

GREEN WAS NOT a team player. He was supremely confident in his own opinion, only rarely referring any of his own cases for a second opinion. Women remained in his care indefinitely. Once, when Green was overseas, one of his patients was referred to me by a member of Green's clinical team for care, but it was already too late. A review of the woman's case records and clinical photographs reveal a great deal about Green's irrational thinking and reasoning, and his approach to the management and welfare of his patients. Phoebe (not her real name) had been under Green's care for 14 years when I first met her in 1976, my first year as a member of the visiting medical staff.

Phoebe was initially referred to the NWH clinic in 1962 with a single episode of bleeding after intercourse. She had had several children and had been widowed for many years; life had not been easy. Phoebe had recently decided to remarry. Bernie Kyle, who saw Phoebe in the clinic, noted that she was overweight, and that there was some 'rawness' in the upper vagina and cervix.[1] He took a smear that reported 'cells strongly suggestive of malignancy'. Her name was placed on the urgent waiting list for an examination under anaesthesia, dilatation of the cervix, curettage, and cone biopsy of the cervix.

As was the custom then, she was admitted two days before the planned surgery. During this time she was assessed by a house surgeon, had routine blood tests and a further cervical smear, which reported 'cells conclusive for malignancy'. Green performed the surgery, noting, like Kyle, that the cervix and upper vagina had an 'unhealthy, granular' appearance, but his notes record 'no suspicion of cancer'. The surgery was uneventful and Phoebe was discharged the following day. Three days later Dr John Sullivan's pathology report recorded a diagnosis of 'carcinoma *in-situ* of the cervix … but the lesion is not extensive'. There was no later supplementary report to suggest that Dr Sullivan had subsequently reviewed the tissue and changed the diagnosis.

Phoebe had smear tests taken at two post-operative visits and both tests were reported as being positive for malignancy. Green wrote, 'I think we will need to review the histology of this patient.' He must have reviewed the slides and changed the diagnosis to a more serious one because three months later he readmitted Phoebe for treatment of invasive cervical cancer.

In 1960 early invasive cervical cancer was treated initially with the application of radium around the tumour, followed by radical hysterectomy. On days of the radium treatments Joan Harbutt, wife of the cancer surgeon, drove to the radiation laboratory at Auckland Hospital, loaded the sealed radium container into the boot of her Morris Minor, delivered it to the operating theatre at NWH (Cornwall) and waited until the radium insertions were completed. On occasions she drove her husband, with the remaining radium, to a private hospital, where Harbutt would treat other women. Finally, she delivered the radium container back to Auckland Hospital and took her husband home for lunch.

At the time of Phoebe's first radium insertion, the operation note (written by Green) records that a review of the slides by Green and Sullivan 'led to a diagnosis of early Stage 1A invasive carcinoma' – the diagnosis had changed from CIS. Following a second radium insertion Phoebe was admitted for a radical hysterectomy. She was discharged from hospital 25 days later, having had four anaesthetics and operations in the previous five months.

Green later stated that he had indeed reviewed the histology with his highly rated pathologist, Dr Sullivan, yet Sullivan made no record of this. In the light of future events it is possible Green reviewed the pathology alone and, influenced by the smear test results, decided to alter the diagnosis. He did not appear to have considered the possibility that the continuing smear abnormalities may have reflected CIS involving the vagina.

Four years after changing the diagnosis to cancer, and treating it as such, Green noted that 'prior to treatment there had been some doubt as to whether the lesion was actually invasive'. Despite the radical treatment, smear abnormalities of variable severity returned and this prompted Green to readmit Phoebe and take four small biopsies from the upper vagina.

These showed the effects of the radium treatment and 'dysplastic epithelium' – an abnormality less serious than CIS. Abnormal smears taken from the severely shortened vagina persisted.

Some years after her initial presentation Phoebe complained to Green of vulval irritation. Green attributed this to intertrigo (benign inflammation) and one can only assume his comments were of reassurance. Some months later Phoebe wrote Green a letter, its cursive handwriting strong and neat.

> The last time I had my check-up was 23.9.65. That is going nearly seven months. Well, when I had my check-up I asked you to examine me in the front, but you said it was nothing, but whatever it is, it is still there. I went to Dr A … and he said it was an ulcer, so I have to bathe it four times a day and put ointment on it. It does not worry me but it does not get better so I would like you to make an appointment for me so I can have you examine me.

Soon after, Phoebe saw Green and he noted 'epithelium on vulva thin and atrophic'. He did not prescribe any treatment and recommended a further visit in one year. Phoebe complained of continued vulval irritation at her next visit in 1967 and Green prescribed hydrocortisone and oestrogen creams for the 'very thin atrophic skin'. Registrars deputised for Green at her next two annual visits and both commented on the abnormality. In 1969 registrar Dr Peter Jennings made the correct clinical diagnosis of 'what appears to be a 4 sq. cm carcinoma *in-situ* lesion on the vulva'.

In 1970, five years after Phoebe first complained of vulval irritation, Green admitted her for examination under anaesthesia, took a biopsy and photographed the lesion (see photo pages). McLean, the pathologist, reported the lesion to be the premalignant lesion carcinoma *in-situ* of the vulva, also called Bowen's disease. Green elected to observe the lesion without treatment. Phoebe continued to have smears, reported as malignant, from the vagina and the vulva.

Although vulval CIS, unlike cervical CIS, is not a common disorder, it was known at the time to be a precancer warranting treatment.[2] Green's decision to photograph, biopsy and *observe* a known cancer precursor without definitive treatment not only placed Phoebe at risk of developing cancer but was outside the terms of his 1966 proposal, which was limited to CIS of the cervix in women under 35. Green clearly felt he had a mandate to observe what happened to untreated CIS of the vulva. His natural history experiment on Phoebe was under way. At that time, removal of the lesion would have been a simple operation.

When Green reviewed Phoebe in 1971 she reported being 'concerned of the red area'. Green noted the lesion to be 'very much larger', now measuring 6 x 4 cm, covering almost the entire left side of the vulva and extending on to the shortened vagina. Phoebe was readmitted the following year, and Green rephotographed the lesion and took two further biopsies, each of which was again reported as vulval CIS. In the operation notes Green commented, 'It may become malignant, but I think she is likely to die of something else long before that.'

Later, Green noted that 'she has been looking with the mirror and [is] somewhat alarmed by what she saw ... she seems a very much more worried and introspective woman than she used to be.' She told Green she blamed her problem on the radiation treatment she had received for cervical cancer. Phoebe declined the offer of a second opinion.

In 1974 Phoebe commented on 'occasional bleeding when she wipes herself'. Green noted 'two elevated areas ... they feel very hard and tough', and that 'the surface is now ulcerated and there has been some further bleeding'. He admitted her in January 1975 for further biopsies and photographs. He observed that 'the whole of the left side of the vulva to within 0.5 cm of the clitoris is now involved in a 'malignant-looking process'. The lesion had also extended to the anal margin and onto the adjacent thigh and vagina. Two biopsies of the vulva and one from the lower vagina were all reported by McLean to be invasive carcinoma. Green's handwritten comment on the pathology report – 'normal chicken wire appearance' – showed he clearly didn't think so. He opined, 'I do not agree with the diagnosis of invasive cancer' – this comment only nine days after he stated it was a 'malignant-looking process'. Green noted that the biopsy sites 'did not heal at all well'.

Soon after, he noted 'a few small patches on the right side of the vulva'. Malignant smears persisted. Phoebe was reviewed by Mr Grieve, who reported, 'This is a slowly progressive invasive lesion ... at her age I would favour a simple vulvectomy and excision of the areas of involved skin on the buttocks. Otherwise treatment should be purely palliative.' Phoebe's daughters were consulted and both declined the offer of surgery for their mother. Over the next 18 months Green reported a 'polypoid mass with a serpiginous outline'. Increasing 'troublesome bleeding' now persuaded Phoebe and her daughters that an operation was becoming necessary. In

Green's absence they were told that surgery would be palliative and made aware of the operative risks.

For almost a decade – and a little over four years since the first biopsy – Green watched a small, symptomatic premalignant condition on the vulval skin extend to cover almost the entire organ, extend to the vagina, anal margins and thigh, and progress to invasive cancer at all these sites. His description of the lesion was that of a cancer, but he did not call it that. By this time Phoebe had had abnormal vaginal smears for 10 years. Green had performed a classic 'natural history' experiment consisting of diagnostic biopsy and observation of the vulval lesion without treatment. In my view this was the last opportunity to treat Phoebe with some possibility of achieving a cure.

Green continued to follow Phoebe with three-monthly outpatient appointments. Early in 1976 he commented on the 'smelly discharge which causes her to have to change three times a day'. A short time later she returned with troublesome bleeding and Green observed 'a hard piece of apparent tumour'. Phoebe and her family now agreed it was time for palliative surgery, although there was a period of further procrastination.

During 1976 Alastair Macfarlane retired and I was appointed as surgeon on C Team with responsibility for the care of women with vulval cancer. In September, while Green was overseas, his colleague Liam Wright asked me to take over Phoebe's management. This had become necessary because of persistent bleeding and increasing anaemia; there was a risk she would bleed to death. I was not convinced the tumour could be resected (cut out) and recommended a preliminary examination under anaesthesia. By now a very large 10 x 8 cm tumour covered the whole of the left side of the vulva, extending into the vagina, onto her left thigh and anal margin. Following this examination I elected to proceed with palliative surgery.

This was a time before CT and MRI scanning, which would have assisted in defining the extent of the cancer. Radiotherapy and chemotherapy were not then considered good initial management options because of severe side-effects and limited benefit. Today, large inoperable vulval cancers are initially treated with chemo-radiation.

Just before the proposed surgery I was approached by Miss Cath Owen, Green's cancer records secretary, a warm, cheerful, motherly woman with a head of thick silver bouffed hair, tinged with blue, which had four or five red HB pencils sticking out of it. Green had established a patient welfare fund to provide amenities such as televisions and comfortable chairs in wards caring for long-term patients. The fund was dependent on donations from grateful patients and their families, and the bring-and-buy stall Miss Owen regularly organised in the hospital foyer. She was also the repository of the collection of photographs Green had taken of Phoebe's vulva; she thought I should have these. These graphic photos illustrate, better than words, the progression of a small, easily operable lesion typical of CIS or Bowen's disease, progressively increasing in size, and finally developing into a large malignant tumour.

Phoebe was admitted for blood transfusions on account of heavy bleeding from the tumour, intermittently requiring a total of 12 units of blood. This forced my hand to proceed with surgery. I performed a posterior exenteration, which included resection of the vagina, the lower bowel, the vulva and the adjacent abnormal skin on the thigh. A general surgical colleague fashioned a colostomy in the abdomen. The surgery was made difficult by scarring and adhesions from her previous radiotherapy and radical hysterectomy. Also, as the surgery was palliative and she was a poor operation risk, we elected not to remove her lymph nodes or to prescribe postoperative radiotherapy. Jock McLean confirmed the previously diagnosed cancers and also reported further cancers on the left side above the clitoris and on the right side of the vulva. Tumour cells were noted to be present in the vaginal edge of the specimen.

Phoebe's convalescence was understandably prolonged: she remained in hospital for nearly three months. When she was discharged her wounds were healed and she was managing her colostomy. I saw her for a single postoperative review one month later. She was living independently and, apart from occasional minor urinary incontinence, appeared to be doing well.

Green, now returned from overseas, determined that her follow-up should be under his care: 'I will attend to her needs in Ward 9.' He brushed me aside when I pointed out to him that earlier removal of the vulval lesion would have prevented the cancer developing. He added, 'You don't have the experience of looking after such cases.' (I didn't.) I have often wondered what would have happened to Phoebe if Green had not gone on overseas leave.

In time Phoebe developed a cancerous lump in the left groin, with a foul-smelling 'chronic discharging sinus'. A little later, malignant ulceration began to occur in the urethral region, necessitating an indwelling catheter. A year after the surgery Green commented, 'As far as I can see nothing [that] has ever been done for this woman's disease has made the slightest difference to its progress, although the vulvectomy saved her from a lot of unpleasant haemorrhage.' Over the next 12 months Phoebe deteriorated inexorably, with haemorrhaging from malignant tissue in her groin, and required further blood transfusions and palliative deep X-ray therapy.

She died three years after her major surgery – from neglect to treat her vulval CIS, 14 years after first presenting with vulval symptoms, and nine years after her first biopsy recorded the presence of a premalignant lesion. During her years under Green's care she had had 46 outpatient attendances, 41 abnormal smear tests, 11 operations and many months in hospital.

Phoebe had been the unwitting victim of Green's natural history experiment – an experiment based on no more than a whim and a misbelief.

It is easy to extend the flawed reasoning Green applied in Phoebe's case to management of the many other women in his experiment. His wilful blindness to the sometimes distressing symptoms, his misinterpretation or dismissal of the findings of the pathology examinations, his unwillingness to consider long-term implications – these factors all contributed to the suffering of his patients and their families.

CHAPTER 7

NINETEEN EIGHTY-FOUR

Herb's study remains the solidest evidence that progression [of carcinoma in-situ*] does occur.*

MONT LIGGINS

MCINDOE WAS BECOMING IMMEASURABLY frustrated: increasing numbers of women were developing cancer and the working party had failed to address the issues he had raised. He had no option – it was time to inform the world. After all, Green had been communicating his version of his study for more than a decade. McIndoe decided to present his analysis of the outcome of Green's experiment to the Third World Congress of the IFCPC in Orlando, Florida, in 1978.

Whereas McIndoe's and McLean's earlier expressions of concern to the medical authorities had been very specific – they had listed details about the women who had developed cancer and those who were of concern – McIndoe's presentation to the congress was a dispassionate, scientific analysis. He did not specifically mention the details of Green's experiment or the management of the women, although he did reference Green's papers. McIndoe simply reported the outcome in 1047 women diagnosed with CIS of the cervix 1955 to 1976 in relation to their follow-up smear results. He reported that cancer had developed in 0.7 per cent of women with normal follow-up smears, and in 16.6 per cent of the women who had abnormal follow-up smears. He concluded: 'There may well have been a different outcome had more active management been undertaken [as a result] of abnormal cytology and colposcopy findings,' adding that 'carcinoma *in-situ* is clearly a disease of consequence.'[1]

McIndoe spoke to what Dr Joe Jordan described as 'a huge turnout', chaired by Professor Dick Mattingly, a distinguished US academic and journal editor. As Jordan observed, 'Ironically 99 per cent of the people in the audience did not realise fully the implications of what [McIndoe] was saying, but those of us like myself, Adolf Stafl [president of the IFCPC] and

Dick Mattingly, who knew the background, were shocked to hear our fears had been founded.[2] Following McIndoe's presentation there were a number of critical questions from the audience suggesting that he should have been more active in treating the women. McIndoe's failure to emphasise that he was describing what had happened to Green's patients, not his own, understandably caused confusion for many in the audience. Malcolm Coppleson sprang to McIndoe's defence, stating it was important to shoot the message, not the messenger.[3]

Similar confusion happened with trainee laboratory technologists. As Michael Churchouse remarked, 'Inevitably new staff would ask, "Why does Prof Green not treat his patients? Why does he let his patients go year after year after we have reported malignancy and not treat them by orthodox means, until eventually some of them progress to invasive cancer?" '[4]

Since there had been no comparable studies of the natural history of CIS of the cervix for almost a generation,[5] the importance of McIndoe's study prompted the editors of two major medical journals to approach him requesting a paper. Professor Hugh Shingleton wrote: '[Your] paper is one of the more important ones presented at the World Congress … we definitely want your work in [a] special issue [of *Obstetric and Gynecologic Survey*].' Mattingly invited McIndoe to submit a paper to the prestigious 'green journal', *Obstetrics and Gynecology*. In Mattingly's view the paper was 'one of the best sources of information on the subject [the natural history of carcinoma *in-situ*] that I know'.[6] He recognised the scientific importance of the new data, and realised he needed to become involved if the information were ever to be published. Over the following years he also became aware of the difficulties facing McIndoe in Auckland and realised that this gentlemanly, reserved but quietly determined non-academic clinician was a small voice in the powerful academic medical hierarchy.

McIndoe discussed his dilemma with McLean and me. Two major medical journals were vying for a scientific paper from an unknown, antipodean gynaecologist. Having an unsolicited paper accepted by one of these journals was an achievement; being invited to contribute was a huge honour. *Obstetrics and Gynecology* was at that time the top-ranked specialist journal in the field, and the obvious choice. McIndoe was excited, and agreed to an abstract being published in *Obstetric and Gynecologic Survey* in 1979.[7] Hindsight proved this to be a wise decision, as almost six years would elapse before our definitive article appeared in print.

Mattingly, who was attending a meeting in Australia in early 1979, elected to visit Auckland en route, 'in the hope that we can have some discussion regarding this paper'.[8] As a matter of courtesy McIndoe discussed Mattingly's forthcoming visit with Green, and a short scientific meeting was arranged, as was customary with international visitors. Green's presentation at this meeting drew heavily on his last article, which had been published five years earlier in the *New Zealand Medical Journal*. In this article Green had concluded that 'the proportion [of cases] progressing to invasion must be small and unlikely to influence favourably incidence and mortality rates'.[9] Using essentially the same material, Green's presentation painted a very different picture to McIndoe's in Florida.

A month after returning home, Mattingly wrote to McIndoe again:

I am writing to remind you of my burning interest to have you complete your study on the long-term results of conservative treatment of cervical intraepithelial neoplasia. This information must reach the scientific press as soon as possible as it may neutralize some of the current interest in this country [the United States] in the cryosurgical treatment of this disease. I know of no other source of information similar to yours with a natural history of this disease so carefully documented.

McIndoe did not respond until December 1980: 'I am sure you understand the unusual situation in which we work. I have had the basic material assembled for some time, but writing is not coming easily, particularly in explaining why so many patients have been left so long with evidence of continuing disease.'

Mattingly responded immediately:

I am sure you know how important this information is in the field of gynecologic oncology and how imperative it is to have this data published as a matter of scientific record. Without publication of your article, this experiment of nature will remain buried in the files of National Women's Hospital. While I fully understand the medical politics involved in collecting the data, I cannot emphasize enough the importance that I and others place on this singular study.

A further eight months elapsed before McIndoe and McLean responded to Mattingly with a draft of an article describing their text as 'still being fluid'. Again Mattingly responded immediately: 'While we were pleased to have this additional information regarding your study, it would be necessary to examine the entire paper before we will be able to completely understand this data. We have been reserving a place for this report in *Obstetrics & Gynecology* for several years, as we are certain that it would be a landmark paper of the natural history of the carcinoma *in-situ*.'

In February 1982 Mattingly told McIndoe how delighted he was to receive the current draft, but

we are still waiting with 'bated' breath for the completion of this landmark report on the natural history of carcinoma in-situ. Since it will soon be four years since we initiated our discussion with you for publishing this material, I am becoming somewhat concerned if the report will ever be completed. As you may recall one of the principal reasons for visiting Auckland in 1979 was to stimulate the early completion of this study. I know of no other source of data as convincing as yours as to the true invasive potential of CIS. I wonder if it would be possible for you and McLean to sit together and realistically discuss this matter and to agree upon a target date for the completion of the study and submission of the manuscript. Would you and McLean consider it advisable to include another author to the paper?

McIndoe, in his reply, again admitted 'writing is not coming easily', providing Mattingly with the usual excuses. He failed to mention one of the more fundamental reasons why he was not making progress: his lack of confidence and constant need for reassurance. In addition his co-author, pathologist Jock McLean, though supportive and encouraging throughout, was neither a scientific writer nor particularly committed to the necessary effort. McIndoe himself had limited medical experience writing for international medical journals.[10] At this point Mattingly suggested 'a further author'.[11]

The warm professional relationship I shared with McIndoe was a mixture of the cautious conservatism and wisdom of age and the enthusiasm of youth. McIndoe had discussed with me his concerns about Green's experiment, and invited me to comment on his scientific writing and on his preliminary drafts of the definitive paper. Now he asked me to join him and McLean, and in June 1982 wrote to Mattingly indicating there would be 'at least one additional author'. 'This will be Dr Ron Jones, a clinician, one of the younger men who will be playing an important part in the management of patients of the gynaecological malignancies in Auckland over the next 20 years or so.'[12]

I accepted the task because I felt that the truth about the experiment and its implications for patients needed to be told. McIndoe and McLean enthusiastically embraced me as their new partner. I set two conditions: first, I needed to verify the evidence as best I could, and this meant our trawling through all the patient records again to familiarise me with the facts; second, I insisted on expert statistical input: the complex management of more than 1000 patients over a lengthy period of time made this a necessity. To that point, McIndoe's analysis was simply in numbers and percentages. I approached Auckland University statistician Peter Mullins, whom I had known when he worked in Bonham's department. McIndoe somewhat reluctantly agreed to this arrangement, but with time he came to appreciate that having a statistician on board enabled us to perform more sophisticated analyses. He also agreed to my suggestion that we should include figures to illustrate abnormal smear tests and surgical interventions: these would provide powerful visual evidence of what had happened to the individual women who developed cancer.

I had heavy commitments as an obstetrician and gynaecologist both at NWH and in the private sector, together with family commitments. When time allowed, McIndoe would come to my home at nights and at weekends and we would work on the paper. We were fully aware of the significance of our endeavours, and the importance of accurate data collection and interpretation. Words, phrases, sentences and paragraphs were discussed, debated, anguished over and rewritten endlessly. It was still the precomputer era and everything was written out by hand. Results were tabulated in pencil so they could be rubbed out and changed as more recent data, such as smear results, became available. The data were recorded in spreadsheet columns on a series of paper sheets taped together and spread across our dining-room table. Handwritten drafts were typed and retyped by McLean's secretary in the pathology department.

On metre-square cardboard sheets McIndoe, in typically obsessive fashion, illustrated the smear and management histories of the women in the experiment who progressed to cancer. Tiny dots represented normal smears, crosses malignant smears, with various other symbols representing differing modes of management. The large board was then photographed and reduced to a size appropriate for publication. Green, who was aware of McIndoe's research, later said he did not update his publications after 1974 because he knew McIndoe was doing so.[13] Green never discussed this with us.

Bonham had learned of McIndoe's 1978 presentation to the IFCPC in Florida during a lecture given by Dr Allan MacLean, a young senior lecturer in obstetrics and gynaecology in Christchurch, at a 1981 meeting of the Waikato Obstetric and Gynaecological Society. Afterwards Bonham, visibly annoyed, had approached MacLean requesting details of the abstract.[14] He was therefore at this point fully aware of the outcome of Green's study – the evidence was available internationally and the results were markedly different from those reported by Green. Inexplicably Bonham still did not act.

In 1982 Professor Harold Fox, the most respected British gynaecological pathologist of his generation, visited NWH at Jock McLean's invitation. We asked him to review a selection of McLean's pathology slides and to comment on a draft of our paper. Over dinner at my home, awash in Fox's favourite Australian shiraz, the air heavily laden with his cigarette smoke, Fox discussed McIndoe's reluctance to implicate directly either Green or the hospital. He was blunt: the hospital had sanctioned Green's experiment; we could not avoid describing and referencing the event. McIndoe was eventually persuaded.

In November 1982 Bonham wrote to Dr Ian Hutchison, the medical superintendent of NWH:

> *I have heard a rumour that Dr McIndoe and possibly another specialist have been reviewing cases of carcinoma in-situ [which] have been managed in the hospital. I have no recollection of approval being given for review of in-situ cases belonging to other consultants and I wonder if they have been reviewing cases, without the approval of the clinicians concerned. This may only be a rumour but I think it may be worthwhile your having a look at it in the first instance because any publication emanating from this hospital must be acceptable to the hospital before it is submitted for publication, as I am sure you will agree.*[15]

There was no policy requiring staff to submit potential publications for approval by hospital authorities. If Bonham's letter was an attempt to silence us and to obstruct the publication, it failed to do so.

In 1982 also, Green retired from the medical school and his hospital appointment. His experiment, however, was not officially stopped until 1988. In that six-year period some of Green's 'followers' continued to manage his patients.

Before our paper was published McIndoe and I attended the Fifth Congress of the IFCPC in Tokyo in 1984, where I presented the final results of our study. In contrast to the response to McIndoe's low-key presentation in Florida six years before, there was a sense of anticipation that this was a significant paper. Coppleson and Jordan had encouraged a large and knowledgeable audience to attend. Aware of the confusion experienced by McIndoe's audience, I made sure I stressed that the high rate of cancer reported in our study was a result of Green's experiment, 'in which a group of women with abnormal smears were managed by limited [diagnostic] biopsy and observation alone.'[16]

In June 1983 Mattingly had critiqued the article, commenting: 'We are still interested in using this paper as a lead article in a forthcoming issue of *Obstetrics and Gynecology*. I do hope that you appreciate the magnitude of our interest in this study and its accuracy.' After we completed further revisions, Mattingly wrote to McIndoe in January 1984: 'We are very anxious to have all of the potential objections to the study recognized and corrected before publication, rather than to continue an on-going debate in the "Letters to the Editor" pages when the study is in print. The publication of your paper is long overdue.'[17] One referee commented:

This is an important paper. Dr Green was the last vocal opponent to the concept of the intraepithelial phase of invasive squamous cell cancer. His unfortunate view[s] received a ready forum at international meetings because it seldom failed to gather a crowd and he remained influential long after an overwhelming body of data made his views untenable. This paper should be the last chapter in the Green saga. The authors are correct in pointing out it will probably be the last large series in which patients with CIS are followed prospectively. Let us hope that is true.[18]

McIndoe wrote to Mattingly in June 1984:

The only significant criticism I have had has been at a clinical level of why some patients were permitted to have continuing undiagnosed abnormal cytology. This was beyond our control … Our statistical data are intended to reinforce the obvious findings that patients with continuing incompletely excised CIS have a much greater chance of subsequent invasive cancer than those in which CIS has been completely excised at the earliest opportunity.[19]

I expressed my own anxieties to McIndoe and McLean: bearing in mind Bonham's earlier attempt to stymie publication, would he try again?' Until we saw the final printed version in the journal in October 1984, we remained anxious about this possibility.

Immediately before publication of 'The invasive potential of carcinoma *in-situ* of the cervix' – ours was the lead article in the issue[20] – McIndoe, McLean and I distributed copies of the paper to members of the senior medical staff. As neither McIndoe nor McLean was keen to present Bonham with his copy, I was given the task, which I carried out with considerable trepidation. I handed it to Bonham saying, 'You should read this and consider the implications.' He received me politely but made no comment.

Following publication, McIndoe discussed the paper with the medical superintendent, Dr Ian Hutchison; later McLean and I discussed the paper with Hutchison's successor, Dr Gabrielle Collison. No doubt both superintendents felt uncomfortable with the message we conveyed. The gist of their response was 'We will have to look into this.' The implication, especially for patients, was very clear to anyone who read the paper.

'There have been,' we wrote,

differences of opinion within the hospital on the invasive potential of carcinoma in-situ *of the cervix. Earlier National Women's Hospital experience pointed to carcinoma* in-situ *having an insignificant invasive potential. In 1966 the senior medical staff agreed to a study of patients whose only abnormal finding was cervical cytology. No further treatment was to be offered to a group of patients … in whom a histologic diagnosis of carcinoma* in-situ *was established by a limited biopsy of the most significant area. The object was to study the natural history of carcinoma* in-situ *of the cervix after a representative biopsy with minimal disturbance of the lesion … The almost universal acceptance of the malignant potential of this lesion has made prospective investigation of the natural history of carcinoma* in-situ *ethically impossible.*[21]

For the purpose of our analysis, we divided all women with CIS into two groups, according to whether they had normal or abnormal follow-up smears following initial management by the hospital's clinicians. Women in Group 1 had normal follow-up smears, indicating they had no sign of disease at that time; Group 2 women had continuing smear abnormalities, indicating CIS was still present. It was most of the women in this second group who formed the basis of Green's natural history study. We emphasised that our 'grouping' was based on smear results, not treatment method ('irrespective of the initial management or the histological completeness of excision'). However, the grouping methodology was misunderstood by some, who assumed that Group 1 women were treated conventionally, while Group 2 were Green's study patients, who received little or no treatment.

We reported that among the 817 Group 1 women (with normal follow-up smears), 12 (1.5 per cent) developed cancer in five to 28 years. We suggested that some were possibly 'new' cancers. In the group of 131 women with persistently abnormal follow-up smears (Group 2), 29 (22 per cent) had developed cancer during follow-up thus far, meaning the risk of developing cancer was 25 times greater in the women who continued to have smear abnormalities (taking follow-up time into account). Additionally, the proportion of women in Group 2 developing cancer increased with time: it was 18 per cent at 10 years, and 36 per cent at 20 years. Combining the numbers across both groupings, the risk that a woman presenting at NWH at that time with CIS would subsequently develop cancer was more than four times greater than in comparable hospitals elsewhere in the world.[22]

Our paper told two stories. First, from a scientific perspective, it described the natural history of CIS of the cervix, confirming evidence that had been accumulating over a century: it would not have surprised many doctors. Second, it detailed the disastrous outcomes for some women from whom treatment was deliberately withheld. This was the story we wanted the staff at the hospital to acknowledge.

The same month our paper was being published in the United States, Auckland's *Metro* magazine published a leading article titled 'The glamorous gynaecologists at National Women's Hospital' about 'the remarkable hospital, its extraordinary research unit and those who toil therein'.[23] These were to be the last effusive comments about the national icon. Soon it would be brought to its knees following exposure of the shocking truth about Green's unethical experiment on a large group of New Zealand women.

CHAPTER 8

ANNUS HORRIBILIS

An in-situ *or an invasive cancer is not necessarily so because McIndoe, McLean and Jones say it is so.*

Herbert Green, 1986

1985 WAS THE MOST indescribably despairing year of my life. My wife was seriously ill, and I sensed the opprobrium of some of my colleagues in response to our paper. Barbara, aged only 43, had developed a breast cancer that had spread to her lymph nodes. We had four children: Helen was 19, Mark 16, Ross 12 and Susan six. The last four years of Barbara's life were punctuated by recurrences of her cancer, requiring repeated treatments with chemotherapy and radiotherapy.

Until something like this happens to you personally, you cannot remotely understand. Of course this happens to millions of others; it is different when it happens to you. To say we were devastated is an understatement. So many words spill off my pen – profound sadness, despair, helplessness, emptiness, weakness. I couldn't run away. I felt angry. What about our future? Why should this happen to us? But then, why shouldn't it? Barbara was incredibly brave and positive; whenever possible her daily routine remained unchanged, and the children's schooling and extracurricular activities were maintained. I continued doctoring. I bitterly regret now that I didn't share my worries, but kept them to myself.

At work I needed to remain a clinical and empathetic doctor. My medical responsibilities provided some distraction from my personal pain, but Barbara's illness and its contingencies constantly simmered in the background. Some of my patients and their families were experiencing the same grief. I wanted to cry out, 'I'm going through the same pain and grief as you are!', but I couldn't. I could empathise, but I could not share my pain.

Immediately after the publication of our paper there was absolutely no response from the academic and senior medical staff of the hospital, or from the wider profession – in particular, from the Royal New Zealand

College of Obstetricians and Gynaecologists. McIndoe, McLean and I were conscious that it was almost certainly being discussed in the hospital – but no one discussed it with us. We knew we were telling an uncomfortable truth, and that our actions contravened the longstanding ethic of loyalty to the hospital and to our senior colleagues. We also knew that, in time, Green, Bonham, even Liggins, and the hospital, might be discredited by what we had written. So it seemed incomprehensible to us that *no one said anything* – not the non-academic medical staff, not the cervical cancer team, not senior members of the university department, and, above all, not Bonham, head of the university department and the man accountable for Green's research.

How could our colleagues apparently ignore the publication, in a prestigious medical journal, of data from their own hospital? Crucially, how could they ignore the fate of the women involved in Green's experiment? The whole gynaecological world had been regularly updated by Green's own papers; his publications constantly underpinned his long-term opposition to cervical screening. Bonham and other staff members knew our 1984 paper contradicted Green's stance – a potentially embarrassing discrepancy within an institution. They must surely have considered the possibility that our findings would eventually raise questions in the wider community.

Why did Professor Bonham and our colleagues fail to discuss their concerns about our paper with us? Power and intimidation breed cowardice: this failure of the senior medical men reflected their lack of courage to confront the truth. Our findings confirmed what they knew to be true. Why else would Bonham and all the other gynaecologists be treating their own CIS patients conventionally, and not simply observing them, as Green was?

However, there were rumours of interest in our work by the recently formed women's health advocacy group Fertility Action.

* * *

In 1985 David Skegg, Professor of Preventive and Social Medicine at Otago University, chaired a working group that published 'Recommendations for Routine Cervical Screening', a blueprint for future screening in New Zealand. As well as stating, 'There is now compelling evidence that cytological screening is an effective preventive measure', it recommended to whom, when and how often such screening should be offered.[1] The executive of the New Zealand Colposcopy Society, Graeme Duncan, Trevor

Svensen and I wrote to the *New Zealand Medical Journal* in 1985 in support of Skegg's paper and referred to the 1984 paper: 'Those who questioned the value of cytology screening and the invasive potential of intraepithelial neoplasia have now been clearly shown to be wrong.'[2] This provoked a letter from Green to the journal, claiming that 'an in-situ or an invasive cancer is not necessarily so because McIndoe, McLean and Jones say it is so'.[3] This was clear evidence Green had read our paper, but he reiterated his view that screening had no effect on cervical cancer mortality. This letter drew Skegg into the correspondence and, in addressing Green's many misconceptions, he coined the phrase 'the unfortunate experiment' to describe Green's study.[4] A number of other authors had already used the word 'unfortunate'.

Dr Murray Jamieson, a former Rhodes Scholar who, it was rumoured, was being considered for head of department on Bonham's retirement, had become head of the cervical cancer team when Green retired. In 1985 he co-authored, with iconoclast Petr Skrabanek, a letter to the *New Zealand Medical Journal* entitled 'Eaten by worms'. Using biblical allusions to sinners it stated: 'True, the victims are not eaten by worms, but gnawed away by cancer (or fear of it). The wages of sex is a positive smear.' The letter argued that there were insufficient deaths to warrant screening.[5] A year later the *Auckland Star* described Jamieson as an opponent of screening, and *More* magazine reported him as saying he 'remain[ed] sceptical about [the screening programme's] effectiveness'.[6] The very unit that should have been promoting cervical cancer prevention was opposing it.

Then in 1987 Bonham, Liggins and Green co-authored an editorial in the *Australian and New Zealand Journal of Obstetrics and Gynaecology* in which they not only cast doubt on the value of cervical screening but emphasised the need to 'seek more objectively the natural history of cervical cancer'.[7] Clearly, our 1984 paper had made no impression on the thinking of the most senior professors at NWH.

The previous year, 1986, I had organised a symposium on 'Cervical cancer and its precursors', sponsored by the Cancer Society and held at the Auckland Medical School. Our paper had at least raised the level of academic awareness of the cervix in the postgraduate department, because Mont Liggins, who had not previously demonstrated any particular interest in this topic, attended. During a discussion on the role of colposcopy he stood up, removed his spectacles and with a theatrical flourish asked the audience, 'Why do you need a colposcope when you have these?'

A number of feminists attended this symposium and took the opportunity to question visiting expert speakers about the nature of CIS. Among them was Sandra Coney, a freelance journalist and a former editor of the feminist magazine *Broadsheet*, who was not afraid to question the status of doctors. As she later wrote,

> ... *I was besieged by National Women's Hospital doctors. One, whom I later learned was Tony Baird, a part-time clinician and ex-superintendent of the hospital, chairman of the New Zealand Medical Association and a very powerful doctor, earnestly told me I was quite wrong. There was no proof, he maintained, that screening would cut down the incidence of the disease [cervical cancer]. When I argued that the evidence from countries like Sweden and Iceland was compelling, he insisted that the facts were open to other interpretations. I pointed out that the 1984 paper showed that untreated CIS will progress to invasion, but he flatly stated that the conclusions of the paper were wrong.*[8]

Yet in 2010 Baird would write, 'I did not read the [1984] paper until the Inquiry [1987] and I recall no discussion about it previously.'[9]

Assuming Sandra Coney to be correct, if Baird did believe that the 1984 paper's conclusions were wrong, he had a moral responsibility to do something about it. In the first instance he could have knocked on my door and discussed his concerns with me. As chairman of the New Zealand Medical Association and a consultant at NWH he was in a strong position to advise and influence senior medical administrators and politicians, and even speak to the media; such actions may have resulted in an independent inquiry being held far earlier than it was. Yet Baird took no action.

* * *

Unbeknown to McIndoe, McLean and me, Sandra Coney and her colleague Phillida Bunkle, a women's studies lecturer at Victoria University, had been informed of our paper as early as 1983. Our statistician, Peter Mullins, had alerted a colleague, Dr Ruth Bonita, who had told Coney and Bunkle. Following publication of our paper, Coney invited Bonita's husband, Professor Robert Beaglehole, a research epidemiologist, to comment on it. On inspecting one of the figures in our paper he immediately pointed out that Green's experiment should have been stopped once the significant discrepancy between the Group 1 and Group 2 women became evident.[10]

Bunkle wrote to Bonham and the other members of the Hospital Ethics Committee asking whether 'the untreated women chose not to have their cancer treated'. Bunkle used the word 'cancer' when she was obviously referring to CIS, but Bonham chose to interpret the question literally and replied that 'none of these patients [has] cancer'. He avoided addressing the issue of consent, and went on to fudge the truth by combining the statistics for the two groups and stating that 'only 4.3% of the patients developed cancer'. He claimed 'the trial was successful' – though, even based on his misleading numbers, this cancer rate was four times that reported in international studies of adequately treated CIS.[11]

Six months later Bunkle rang McIndoe, who reluctantly discussed our paper with her. He told her it was published in order 'to get it out in the open. We didn't want to be vindictive. We wanted his [Green's] peers to judge.' McIndoe later observed that despite unsuccessful efforts in the mid-1970s to get the study stopped 'it never ended. Green carried on with his varied management to the end of his days.' He also said, 'Green's management is being repeated by doctors who are Green's followers.'[12]

In April 1985 I received a letter from a Jackie McAuliffe from Fertility Action, asking me to 'clarify some points' in the 1984 article.[13] Her questions were confused and not able to be answered as they were presented. Also, my personal crisis was intense at the time so I directed her to McIndoe. According to Coney, McIndoe's 'tetchy' reply said Fertility Action had failed to understand how the data had been analysed, and that answers to their questions were impossible. Coney believed McIndoe's response 'seemed very evasive, reinforcing our suspicion at the time … [that] the authors themselves had something to hide'. However, Coney later acknowledged that 'when this letter [from McAuliffe] was composed we didn't realise … we had made mistakes in our reading' of the report. Like Green's supporters some years later, they had failed to appreciate that the two groups of women we described were established on the basis of positive or negative follow-up smears, reflecting cure or persistent disease – irrespective of the type of initial treatment. They had also wrongly concluded that we, the authors, were ourselves involved in the study and were thus merely writing up our own results.[14]

Fertility Action continued to investigate the background to our paper, then unexpectedly they had a 'real breakthrough'.[15] A woman who had been a patient of Green for many years, and who had recently been treated for cervical cancer, contacted them. Clare Matheson, then a secondary school teacher, had been referred to Green's NWH clinic late in 1964 with a smear abnormality, and a diagnosis of CIS was established soon after: Green had included her in his experiment more than a year before he had gained approval for it. Over succeeding years he made no attempt to eradicate her lesion. She was discharged in 1979 following some normal smears, but by then her cervix was so badly scarred following multiple diagnostic biopsies that it was impossible to take a good smear. By this time she had visited the clinic on 34 occasions, had 31 smears (24 abnormal), 10 colposcopies, six biopsies, and five operations under general anaesthesia. Some biopsies had even reported 'microinvasive' cancer and the most recent 'carcinoma devoid of underlying stroma – probably carcinoma *in-situ*'. At one point, fed up with constantly attending the clinic, Matheson intimated to Green that he should get someone else to be his guinea pig. '"You'll do as you are told," he said loudly, his face flushed with anger.'[16]

In his discharge letter to Matheson's general practitioner in 1979 Green wrote, 'I do not think she needs to attend the clinic for further follow-up as she has no more chance than the next person of now developing any carcinoma of the cervix.' Following her discharge, Matheson's doctor failed to take further smears for six years until late in 1988, when she presented to him with abnormal bleeding. A smear taken at the time was abnormal and she was referred to a private gynaecologist, Dr Graeme Overton, with a summary of her NWH records. He told her he would have performed a hysterectomy 15 years earlier, as she had been 'left sitting on a time bomb'. Although, in Matheson's words, Overton was 'obviously disgusted and angry at my condition' and 'totally disagreed with the way Green had treated [me]', his later referral letter to the hospital was ambiguous – 'Mrs Matheson was a little upset that this carcinoma has developed after she had been followed at NWH for such a long time ... but I have not discussed in detail with her whether that was good or bad management.'[17] Overton was unable to get a clear view of her cervix because of the distorted anatomy resulting from her previous surgeries. A further biopsy performed under anaesthesia confirmed invasive cervical cancer and Clare was treated at NWH with radioactive caesium and a radical hysterectomy. Fortunately she remains alive and well.

In a cruel irony, Matheson's general practitioner, who had been assured by Green that his patient was at no increased risk of cancer, was charged by the Medical Practitioners' Disciplinary Tribunal and found guilty of failing to take cervical smears following her discharge from NWH. The tribunal recorded mitigating factors, including Green's discharge letter. One needs, perhaps, to feel some sympathy for the accused GP. He certainly should have been taking smears but he could not have been expected to be familiar with the extent and implications of Matheson's mismanagement by Green. A further irony was that the Disciplinary Tribunal called as a witness Green's replacement, Dr Murray Jamieson, a man also described as 'an opponent of cervical screening'.

* * *

The term 'whistle-blower' was not in common use in the 1980s. McIndoe, McLean and I had seen our role merely as telling the truth: we considered it our duty to inform the medical profession of our conclusions relating to Green's experiment. Bonham, Green and the hospital authorities had ignored almost 20 years of written concerns, but we were convinced the international publication of our paper would result in definitive action. As McIndoe suggested, the issue (Green's experiment) could, we hoped, be resolved by the profession at a local level without too much fuss.

People have asked me since why we did not go to the media. But in those days doctors on the lower rungs of the medical hierarchy would never have dreamt of doing such a thing. We did not even consider approaching the Medical Council, whose vice-chairman, Bruce Grieve, was a senior NWH gynaecologist who had supported Green from the outset. But Coney and Bunkle had other ideas, and they soon set about gathering information for their forthcoming article in *Metro*. Clare Matheson became 'Ruth', the unfortunate patient in their story. This was manna from heaven for feminist health activists – elderly male gynaecologists experimenting on women without their knowledge or consent. They quickly assembled a team of medical advisers, lawyers and supporters to assist them.

The next step for Coney and Bunkle was to interview the people directly involved in the experiment – Bonham and Green – and those of us who reported the outcome, although I declined because at that time I was a member of the Auckland Hospital Board Investigations Committee. Coney's book, *The Unfortunate Experiment*, documents those meetings. Bonham was courteous during their two-hour interview, but his answers were elusive, employing innuendo, especially when referring to our 1984 paper. Coney observed that he rarely used frank statements and had a tendency to circumlocution. He denied that he was against cervical screening and insisted that Green's experiment was not to study the natural history of CIS. When Bonham was asked who could have stopped the experiment, he named Green, the medical superintendent and the Hospital Medical Committee, but not himself. He then went on to say the study was not terminated but 'became general treatment'.

In short, he placed all the blame on others – for example, 'the colposcopic service was not good enough', implicating McIndoe. My good friend and valued colleague Bill McIndoe had died suddenly the previous year from a heart condition. He could not defend himself. Bonham did not criticise Green, however, describing him as a 'unique sort of free thinker'.

Understandably, Green himself was very defensive when interviewed by Coney and Bunkle. David Skegg came in for heavy criticism from Green, particularly for his phrase 'the unfortunate experiment'. Green disputed the findings of the 1984 paper, using his well-established ploy against pathology – 'just because McLean says they are invasive does not mean they are'.

Jock McLean was happy to be interviewed. Coney and Bunkle may have attempted to loosen him up with a bottle of wine, but he remained circumspect yet frank, describing the background to Green's experiment, and his and McIndoe's attempts to stop it. Regarding the forthcoming publicity, he said, 'I don't give a damn, but we don't want to bring [the hospital] into disrepute.'[18] Having created this crisis, we were concerned about the rehabilitation of our hospital.

McIndoe's daughter, Mary Whaley, was privy to her father's telephone conversation with Coney about our 1984 paper. When Mary told him he 'had been a bit mean', McIndoe said he 'was testing her [Coney] to see if he could trust her and whether she had any gravitas and integrity', but also said he felt excited that 'something might happen'. 'Following Dad's death,' Mary explained, 'Bunkle wrote to Mum expressing her sympathy and adding that she was sorry "they hadn't finished their research". The letter intimated that Bonham had suggested Green's experiment was Dad's experiment; this was the last straw!'[19]

Noeline McIndoe and Mary discussed Bunkle's letter with me. We sorted through his papers – gathered together all the notes, memoranda and correspondence dating back two decades relating to Green's experiment, copied them, and Mary took them to Sandra Coney. According to Coney these were 'the final pieces of the jigsaw'.[20]

Back in 1981 McIndoe had encouraged me to accompany him to the 4th World Congress of the International Federation of Cervical Pathology and Colposcopy in London, and suggested that I present a scientific paper. This was excellent advice: I had to research, prepare and present a paper to an international audience. I took as my subject the natural history of CIS of the vulva – an uncommon condition, but increasingly frequent in younger women. I hadn't forgotten Phoebe: was she part of a usual pattern or was her cancer a rare sequel? I had reviewed all documented cases of vulval CIS cases at NWH, identifying 23 cases over the preceding 21 years.[21] Four of them, all managed by Green, had had only a biopsy and all had progressed to invasive cancer within eight years. Phoebe was one of them.

Now, in 1986, buoyed by the scientific success of the 1984 paper, McLean and I published a definitive paper on the natural history of CIS of the vulva – again in *Obstetrics and Gynecology*. By now there were 36 cases. We referenced Green and stated that 'this conservative approach [was] an extension of a study of the conservative management of carcinoma *in-situ* of the cervix'. We concluded that 'the untreated lesion in women in middle and later life has a significant invasive potential'.[22] While this was being published, Coney and Bunkle were putting the finishing touches to their forthcoming *Metro* article.

The fuse that began smouldering after publication of our 1984 paper, then burned more brightly with the 1986 paper, burst into flame when *Metro* published 'An unfortunate experiment' in June 1987.

CHAPTER 9

IRRECONCILABLE DIFFERENCES

The meeting closed in a happy haze of goodwill, but we were all fully aware of where our loyalties were meant to lie.

MICHAEL CHURCHOUSE

RUMOURS THAT A FORTHCOMING exposé of Green's experiment was to feature in Auckland's *Metro* magazine circulated for some months before it was published in June 1987.[1] Sandra Coney and Phillida Bunkle had certainly done their homework. The story of Green's 'unfortunate experiment' was a shocking revelation. How could this be happening in NWH – the hospital where many *Metro* readers were born or had given birth?

The central themes of the *Metro* article were our 1984 paper, and 'Ruth', a subject in Green's experiment, who had inadequately treated CIS and subsequently developed cancer. The story was bolstered by interviews with a number of key figures, including Green, Bonham, McIndoe and McLean. I considered their article to be a reasonably fair and balanced account. Their only mistake was to comment that Group 1 patients had had treatment with conventional techniques, and normal smears, and this error has been perpetuated in subsequent revisionism.[2] Later, Coney stated that she 'over-simplified the division of women' for the convenience of readers.[3] However, Coney and Bunkle's message was clear – Green had performed an unethical experiment on a large group of unsuspecting women with a known precancerous condition. Many went on to develop cancer; some others were probably still at risk.

With the exception of Jock McLean and Ian Ronayne, no one on the NWH medical staff discussed the *Metro* article with me after it was published. No doubt the senior members of the academic staff were shocked and upset by it, and many of the staff – doctors, nurses and others – would have been unhappy to see their hospital and senior colleagues vilified in the media. However, human nature being what it is, some staff who had crossed swords with Bonham or Green may have felt these two men were receiving their comeuppance.

As Coney observed, there was no immediate response to the *Metro* article – 'the media wouldn't initially touch the thing with a barge pole',[4] but the issue was soon raised by the Auckland Hospital Board. The chairman, Sir Frank Rutter, said a report was being prepared, and Dr Leslie Honeyman, the Auckland Hospital Board's medical superintendent-in-chief, recommended to the board: '… on the basis of the [*Metro*] article, and information subsequently obtained, I am of the opinion that full investigation both of the historical origins of these concerns, and of present day practice and procedure is required.'[5] In 1986, when a doctor outside NWH had drawn his attention to our paper and the potential ethical ramifications of Green's study, Honeyman had become the third medical superintendent-in-chief who failed to intervene.[6]

Soon the public outcry in the wake of the *Metro* article was more than the board could handle, and members quickly requested the minister of health to establish an official inquiry.

* * *

The title of the inquiry and its final report, *Allegations Concerning the Treatment of Cervical Cancer at National Women's Hospital and into Other Related Matters*, was misleading.[7] No one ever suggested there were any issues relating to the treatment of cervical *cancer* (apart from microinvasive cancer) at NWH; the central issue was the failure to treat the precancer, CIS. This has continued to cause confusion to this day. The words 'carcinoma *in-situ*' do, however, appear in small print in the body of the Public Notice. The inquiry was to be headed by Auckland Family Court judge Silvia Cartwright. On 10 June 1987 Minister of Health Michael Bassett announced that she would run 'a short, sharp Ministerial Inquiry which was not to be a witch-hunt or circus'.[8]

Following the evening television announcement, an angry colleague knocked on my door. His face was flushed and he was obviously very agitated. I invited him into our kitchen, where Barbara was sitting. He came straight to the point. 'You have caused all this trouble. This is the most irresponsible and reprehensible act I have encountered in my entire life. We will show your paper is totally wrong. At least this inquiry will sort out the truth.'

I felt my blood pressure rising.

He continued, 'Have you given any thought to how Professors Bonham and Green and their families feel at this time?'

Barbara burst into tears. He put his hand on her shoulder and said, 'Dear, dear, it's not your fault.'

This momentary distraction gave me an opportunity to collect my thoughts. 'Have you given any thought to the victims of the experiment – the women, most of whom are married with husbands and families?' I was perhaps thinking of my own family at that moment: Barbara was shortly to begin a further course of treatment.

He reiterated, 'We will prove you wrong and you will be discredited.'

The confrontation was brief, a clash between an advocate for the women and an advocate for the doctors facing a public inquiry. He quickly left our house. Barbara and I hugged and shared our tears.

When I arrived at NWH the Monday following the announcement of the inquiry, I learned all too soon the meaning of the phrase 'persona non grata'. The usual friendly morning exchanges with my colleagues were replaced by a coolness that sent a very clear message. Some avoided me, some offered cursory greetings and some looked at me askance. Conversations stopped when I entered a ward office or approached a group discussion in a corridor. McLean was lucky, he could shut himself in his basement laboratory office, but I had my clinical duties in the hospital wards and theatres; I had not considered this scenario when I agreed to assist in writing the paper. I was a broken man, but I could not run away; I knew I had to face up to whatever lay ahead. The only comfort was that I knew we had described the truth as best we could and, come what may, we could defend our findings. I was conscious of the spirit of McIndoe at my shoulder. However, I was poorly equipped to deal with what lay ahead.

Tony Baird defended Green, telling the media that there were many 'slurs and inaccuracies' in the *Metro* article, that the accusations were wrong, that the inquiry would clear Green and the hospital and that, in most cases, the women had been given the best available treatment.[9] Colin Mantell, a professor at NWH who had not previously been involved in the saga, tried to put together a consensus statement for the media on behalf of all hospital medical staff, in order to heal the divisions and tensions that had developed within the hospital and the consequent lack of morale. This proved impossible.

It soon became evident there were four factions at NWH: McLean and me; Kyle and Ronayne, who were privately supportive; Green, Bonham and their supporters, including the medical superintendent, Dr Gabrielle Collison; and the rest, who did not want to become involved. This last group no doubt spent much time in offices and corridors grumbling about the unfairness of it all. I would like to believe some of them privately supported McLean and me, but it is impossible to know.

Three Auckland Hospital Board medical superintendents-in-chief and two NWH superintendents had been aware of concerns about Green's experiment and up to this point had chosen to hide behind their bureaucratic cloaks, as if to say, 'We are not clinicians and so we are not in a position to comment on clinical matters.' All knew – if not from their medical training, at least from the extensive publicity – of the significance of smear tests in cancer prevention. These people had a public responsibility for community health and should have become involved. Above all, they had a responsibility to consider the welfare of the women in Green's experiment.

Collison, relatively new to NWH, was understandably keen to demonstrate her loyalty to staff. Michael Churchouse remembered when she 'surprised us by announcing she was going to grace the cytology staff's afternoon tea time with a visit'.

This was an unprecedented event indeed and we made sure there was a full attendance in our tiny tearoom. Of course we did not, at that time, connect her visit with the Inquiry into Prof Green's experiment.

Gabrielle drank her coffee and charmingly discoursed on how the medical staff must stick together and not make statements which might discredit the hospital. She used words like 'loyalty' and 'misunderstanding' …
I could hardly believe my ears.

The meeting closed in a happy haze of goodwill, but we were all fully aware of where our loyalties were meant to lie.[10]

Divisions were present not only among the NWH doctors but also among members of the Auckland District Health Board – between the elected representatives and the bureaucrats. Elected representatives were told by their executive that, under existing hospital board regulations, members were 'vicariously liable' for an employee's actions and they should not comment.[11] Dr Peter Davis challenged the manner in which the board executive handled the crisis, but chairman Sir Frank Rutter used his casting vote to delay discussion of a statement tabled by Davis. Davis expressed his concern: 'All this has occurred in my name but without my concurrence. At no stage have I, as an elected member, been consulted, advised or briefed on any but the most peripheral aspects of the Board's legal representation before the Inquiry.'[12] Matters were further complicated because the deputy chairman of the board, Judith Bassett, was the wife of Health Minister Michael Bassett, and Peter Davis was the husband of Helen Clark, who soon succeeded Bassett as health minister.

It appeared to McLean and me, as the various players began to assemble their legal teams for the inquiry, that the defence of NWH was going to be seen as paramount and that we were expendable. No member of the senior medical staff, including Collison, discussed issues relating to the forthcoming inquiry with us, or supported us before, during or after the inquiry. I fail to understand those of my colleagues who continued to support Green, when all of them treated CIS in their own patients, knowing it was a cancer precursor.

Green spoke confidently to the media, offering his favourite phrase – 'my conscience is quite clear' – to the *Sunday Star*, and similarly telling the *New Zealand Herald*, 'My secret weapon is my conscience – it is absolutely clear.'[13] Green's conscience is at the heart of this story.

On the eve of the inquiry, with some trepidation I decided to talk with Bonham. I knew it was not in Green's nature to admit he might be wrong, but I thought Bonham might be having second thoughts. In my short prepared speech I told him I was confident our 1984 paper would stand up to the scrutiny of the inquiry. In the light of events, would he regard Green's study as misguided, admit fault and consider apologising? Bonham listened and thanked me. I left. It was too late: he was already caught in Green's web and lawyers were now involved.

I had previously alerted Hugh Rennie, lead barrister for the Medical Protection Society (who represented the McIndoe estate, McLean and myself at the inquiry), to potential issues arising from our paper, so he was not surprised when I phoned him and asked for his legal advice. Naively I had thought this 'short, sharp inquiry' advocated by Bassett would be chaired by a lawyer and would involve Green and Bonham, Coney and Bunkle, and independent medical experts who would verify the facts in the *Metro* article and our paper and produce reports. Rennie quickly disabused me of these thoughts, leaving me in no doubt that it would be indeed be a 'witch-hunt and a [media] circus'. How right he was about the media circus.

An urgent meeting was arranged for McLean and me with Hugh Rennie, Chris Hodson and Jane Lovell-Smith, lawyers for the Medical Protection Society. They needed to do a thorough assessment of the credibility of their clients in relation to the issues to be brought before the inquiry. After some amiable small-talk Rennie, in a characteristically understated way, took an unexpected tack: he implied that McLean and I might have had some shortcomings we wished to reveal. How did we know our 1984 paper was factually correct? Could we defend it?

His innuendoes upset me and I burst out angrily, 'They created the problem – not us!'

A smile spread slowly over Rennie's face. 'Just testing,' he replied laconically.

McLean and I had not realised we were to be put under the microscope. Just before the inquiry I attended a meeting in Queensland of the Australian Society for Cervical Pathology and Colposcopy. To my complete surprise on the first morning I ran into Hodson and Lovell-Smith.

'Are you here to check up on me?' I asked.

Hodson demurred. 'We're here to learn something of the subject.'

I introduced them to Professor Malcolm Coppleson and they discussed Green's experiment and the forthcoming inquiry.

I have no doubt they were, at least in part, using this international audience to assess my credibility, while at the same time elucidating for themselves past and present opinions on the nature of CIS of the cervix and its management. Without exception all the experts at the meeting would have confirmed that CIS was a precancer and should be treated. How ironic that a couple of lawyers, who barely knew where a cervix was, would take the trouble to attend such a meeting, while Professor Herb Green, New Zealand's expert on the subject, had never become involved in this active trans-Tasman specialist medical society. Hodson and Lovell-Smith were the only inquiry counsel to attend the meeting.

McLean was the next to be tested. Early in the inquiry Bonham had approached Rennie to say that McLean's pathology was 'wrong', as was our paper, and he was sure the authors would be discredited – almost identical words to those said by my colleague on the evening the inquiry was announced. This was of some concern because in recent years McLean had had a number of health problems. Our case rested on the quality of

McLean's pathology. If this should come into question, so would our paper, and the lawyers needed urgent confirmation on this point.

During these enquiries one name constantly came up: Professor Ralph Richart, from the Columbia Presbyterian Hospital in New York. He was the man who had coined the new term cervical intraepithelial neoplasia (CIN) to replace the older terms dysplasia and carcinoma *in-situ*. We later learned he had given Coney and Bunkle advice during the writing of their article. He was happy to appear pro bono for us as an expert witness, providing it was during his academic holiday and the Medical Protection Society paid his expenses.

I recall the palpable tension in McLean's laboratory office when Richart began to review a selection of histology slides. Would he confirm McLean's diagnoses of CIS? Happily there were no concerns. Richart did differ with McLean regarding some of his diagnoses of CIS with microinvasion, but noted that internationally respected pathologists frequently debated this particular diagnosis. Both McLean and I had passed our pre-inquiry tests. Despite our concerns about McLean's health, his evidence to the inquiry was refreshingly honest. In his words, 'I don't give a toss what the National Women's staff think about me.'[14] One opposition counsel suggested that Richart's opinions would be valued only if his opinion supported McLean. This comment angered Rennie since it demonstrated that the Green camp regarded the inquiry as a legal litigation situation rather than an inquiry set up to establish the truth.[15]

By the time the commission was established, battle lines had already been drawn in the hospital. Bonham – far from accepting my suggestion that he admit fault, apologise and assist in rectifying the problem – had, along with the senior medical staff, and university and hospital administrators, decided to defend the allegations. Naturally I was excluded from these discussions.

At the time of the inquiry, McLean and I kept our distance from the Coney–Bunkle team, regarding them with some suspicion and reservation. If the whistle-blowers had joined forces with the feminists, our professional futures in Auckland would have been untenable. But over time we came to appreciate that we were on the same side.

* * *

The inquiry, which began on 18 June 1987, was a bonanza for those in the law and the media. Rows of dark-suited lawyers, young and old, filled the front half of the large government office where the inquiry was held: Silvia Cartwright deplored their 'jockeying for position'.[16] TV cameras and reporters were positioned along one side. Separate legal teams represented the various parties to the inquiry – Coney and Bunkle, Green and Bonham, the Auckland Hospital Board, the University of Auckland, the Cancer Society, the New Zealand Medical Association, and us. The back half of the room was reserved for the public.

Bassett's early prediction of a 'short, sharp inquiry' soon proved to be wide of the mark: it ran for 68 days over the next six months and featured regularly on national television.

Although the stated purpose of the inquiry was to establish the truth and not to run a trial, the presence of Coney, Bunkle and their lawyers in the front row gave the appearance of a 'prosecution' team – a team led by Dr Rodney Harrison and financed by the government. Harrison sought unsuccessfully to have the inquiry apportion blame or responsibility. In Cartwright's opinion, 'the question of culpability would not assist in the overall determination of where the best path lay in the future'. From the beginning she made it clear that the inquiry was to be inquisitorial, a fact-finding mission to investigate and then report on its findings. Yet she observed, 'The very nature of the issues under investigation and the considerable interest evinced by various factions combined to create a more adversarial atmosphere.'[17]

Plucked from the relative obscurity of the Family Court to lead what was to become New Zealand's most important and far-reaching medical inquiry, Silvia Cartwright faced an enormous challenge. As she explained, 'I conducted the inquiry as a feminist and lawyer ... I could see it wasn't just about disease, it was about these women's whole lives and families.'[18] Cartwright would have been familiar with the positive media hype that had long surrounded NWH and aware, too, of the international acclaim in the obstetric field of Sir William Liley and Graham (Mont) Liggins, both close personal friends of Green. She would have been conscious, too, that the medical profession was critically examining her performance. Her grace and composure throughout were remarkable.

The judge recognised the need for readily accessible, trustworthy and re-spected medical advisers who were independent of the University of Auck-land. The commission appointed Professor Eric MacKay, a Brisbane gy-naecologist with a special interest in cancer; Dr Charlotte Paul, a medical epidemiologist from the University of Otago; and Dr Linda Holloway, a pathologist, also from Otago. Cartwright familiarised herself with all aspects of the case. She read widely; she spoke with nurses; she visited colposcopy clinics; she learned about relevant techniques such as cytology; and, most importantly, she encouraged women to talk to her. 'How impressed I was,' she wrote, 'with the courage and determination of the [75] women who came to speak with me, a stranger to them, and with their willingness to talk about such a personal and, in many instances, distressing part of their lives.'[19]

Our papers and the *Metro* article provided only one side of the story. Was Green being unfairly condemned? Was his 'conservative approach' in fact saving women from unnecessary surgery, as he claimed? Cartwright knew she needed to examine both sides of the argument fairly and, as far as possible, to arrive at the truth. To her credit her report was never challenged in the courts, as had happened with the 1981 Mahon report on the Erebus tragedy. It cannot be stressed sufficiently that the final report of the inquiry was *not* based on either our paper or the *Metro* article. It was based on the evidence of expert witnesses, independent examination of patient records, and analyses by the expert advisers using all the material available to them.

Green's lawyer, David Collins, a young, fresh-faced barrister, was faced with a monumental assignment. His client, a well-known professor, was accused of experimenting, without their knowledge or consent, on women with an easily treatable, but potentially lethal, precancerous condition. Once Collins had thoroughly researched the case and interviewed Green extensively he would soon have realised that presenting his client in the best possible light would be a formidable undertaking. Green's intransigence made it difficult for Collins to make a case for him and as I watched I was left with the impression that the lawyer had little option but to do his best to follow the script Green had written for him.

No one knows how many individual supporters Green and his lawyer tried to assemble on his behalf. I am aware that Green's wife, Joan, contacted some of his colleagues who declined to support him in the witness box. Green hoped desperately that his close friend and colleague Mont Liggins would appear for him but, although Liggins' name remained on the commission noticeboard throughout the inquiry, and he did submit a brief of evidence supporting Green, he remained overseas until the inquiry was over. Another Green ally, Bill Liley, had committed suicide in 1983.

* * *

The first matter to be dealt with at the inquiry was patient files. Judge Cartwright requested that all files referred to in our 1984 paper be made available to the commission. The Auckland Hospital Board's lawyers tried to prevent this, claiming medical privilege and pleading lack of staff, but a ministerial notice in the *New Zealand Gazette* overcame this impasse. Then David Morris, the colourful, aggressive Hospital Board lawyer, objected to Coney and Bunkle having access to patient files. This, too, was resolved.

The hearing began with submissions from Coney and Bunkle, followed by Green assisted by his counsel. Coney's exhausting four-day sojourn in the witness box set the scene for the rest of the inquiry.

Collins opened Green's defence with one of his client's favourite quotes: 'We have first raised a dust and then complain we cannot see.'[20] He said he hoped Green's evidence would settle the dust storm caused by the misunderstanding: the 'so called conservative treatment programme for women with carcinoma *in-situ* was designed to cure them with a minimum degree of surgery – there was never any intention not to cure them'. He went on to say that the programme of treatment did not infringe medical ethics or come close to human experimentation, and that 'Dr Green's evidence would be a challenge for some'. Finally, he said Green's evidence would prove to be a 'fortunate experience' for NWH.[21]

In fact by the time of the inquiry in 1987 Green had largely lost interest in the natural history of CIS of the cervix. Seventeen years had elapsed since his last international publication and 13 years since his last New Zealand publication on the subject. In 1980, 18 months before his retirement, he took nine months' sabbatical leave. In his report to the University of Auckland he admitted his 'long continued interest in the epidemiology and natural history of the common female malignancy, cancer of the cervix … is now only a minor one'.[22] (His focus by this time was royal births.)

In the witness box Green was variously described as 'a bewildered old man' and 'a draught horse with blinkers on'.[23] Certainly he looked older than his 71 years, and many felt sorry this elderly man had to endure more than a week in the witness box. To his credit, Green faced his accusers bravely. His written evidence and responses during cross-examination were similar in style to his recorded writings and verbal expressions over the preceding quarter-century. He rarely answered a question directly. The inquiry revealed the complexity of Green's character: on the one hand his deliberate obfuscation, on the other, an often benevolent approach to the women under his care.

Those present at the inquiry confronted the same difficulties that McIndoe and McLean had encountered over the years. Green claimed his management was not an 'unfortunate experiment' but a 'very fortunate programme' because it had avoided unnecessary surgery. He was 'acutely conscious' that some women had died, but they did not die as a consequence of the treatment they received at NWH. He had reread the confirmed minutes of the 1966 Senior Medical Staff meeting, which had been recorded by a layperson, and extraordinarily he now stated he did not agree with them: 'I did not say my aim was to prove that carcinoma *in-situ* was not a premalignant disease.'[24]

On occasions Green patronised his questioners. Responding to a question about his approach to treatment, he replied, 'Geheimrat.' Cartwright said, 'I think you had better interpret: I'm struggling a little here, Dr Green.' Green replied that it was 'a name for an old German professor-type who was the big boss and nobody could do anything without letting [him] know ...' When questioned about his 'special series', he replied, 'Special series has a particular meaning in a medical context that I cannot expect you to understand.' When challenged by claims he had made about inaccuracies in the *Metro* article he said, 'The words are wrong. I certainly deny I said them.' When a recording of his words was produced, Green had to concede his recollection had been incorrect.

He dismissed our 1984 and 1986 papers with the same argument he had used over the years: 'Those so-called premalignant lesions which [are] cured would never have become malignant if left alone, while the lesions that are truly premalignant are not curable by excision.'[25] When invited to comment on his skills in the four fields represented by the authors of the 1984 paper – colposcopy, pathology, gynaecology and statistics – he stated that his experience was greater than our 'collective assessment'. Questioned about his qualifications in pathology he said, 'I think my experience would be the same as many formally trained pathologists.' And when asked about the ethics of a proposed study by the noted British epidemiologist Archie Cochrane, a study similar to his own, Green responded, 'Even I [in 1970] was dubious about the ethicality of such a trial because cytology screening and the theory of every invasive cancer starting from carcinoma *in-situ* was too well established and I wasn't surprised it was turned down by the [British] Medical Research Council.' Hugh Rennie then asked him, 'The British Medical Research Council considered such a trial unethical in 1970 but you continued yours for some years?' Green replied, 'Cochrane's trial was different.'[26]

At the inquiry, doctors accustomed to being in private, collegial hospital meetings were placed before a professional coterie of barristers in a public forum. Lawyers trade in words. Witnesses are often asked to clarify or comment on the use of particular words or phrases; sometimes lawyers shape questions in order to confuse witnesses. Green was under considerable stress in the witness box and at times he clearly became confused. A headline, '"Questions misled me", says Green', was correct.[27] Then he mistakenly blundered into suggesting that the word 'invariably' should have been included in his 1966 study proposal. This, of course, only made matters worse. As David Skegg observed, in order to test that CIS did not 'invariably' progress to cancer would involve continuing the study until every woman developed cancer.[28] Green was not alone in this semantic conundrum; later in evidence both Faris and Bonham were lured into the same mistake.

Newspapers delighted in the personal comments that surfaced during the course of the inquiry. A former nurse described Green's enthusiasm for smear tests: 'A woman could hardly get past the appointment counter without having her pants off and a smear taken.' She also described him as 'one of the first feminists'. A colleague described how Green gave hope to the terminally ill, and of how he wished he had been able to care for his terminally ill mother. Naturally Green was upset by the headline 'Some are calling me a murderer'.[29]

Having spent most of his time in the witness box defending the notion that biopsy was treatment, and arguing that there was no research programme, Green finally conceded that there was a research programme into the natural history of CIS and he believed it had continued since his retirement six years earlier. He said the late Dr Wilton Henley, medical superintendent-in-chief at the time, had described it perfectly as 'clinical cartography'. He also conceded there was a risk of cancer being overlooked at the beginning of his study but still maintained that 'less than 10%, and [maybe even] less than 5% of carcinoma *in-situ* would progress to invasion'.[30]

No one learned anything new from Green's time in the witness box: his testimony in the end confirmed what he had always believed and expounded. After eight exhausting days he was admitted to Greenlane Hospital with a chest infection. Forty-three days into the inquiry Green's

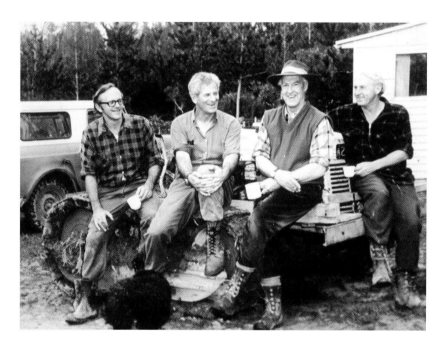

Friends on a crawler, mid-1970s. *Left to right*: Mont Liggins, John Groome
(forestry adviser), Herb Green, Bill Liley.

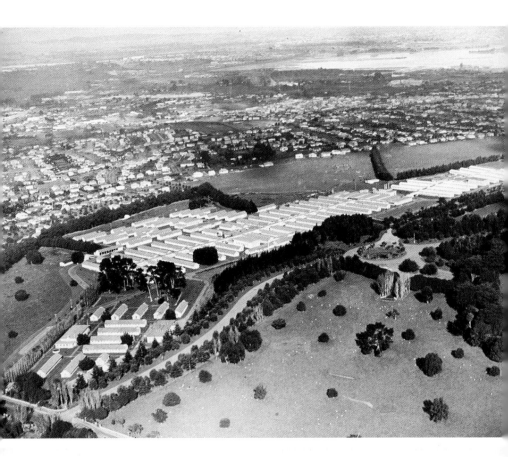

Aerial view of the US Army 39th General Hospital, Cornwall Park, Auckland, 1944. The Cornwall Hospital Obstetric and Gynaecological Unit was located in part of this complex.

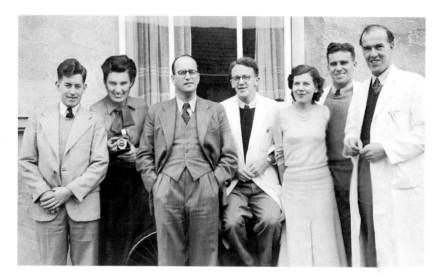

Resident medical staff, Cornwall Hospital Obstetric and Gynaecological Unit, 1948. *Left to right*: David Cross, Helen Borg, Algar Warren, Mont Liggins, Lindsay Johnson, Bob Gudex and Herb Green.

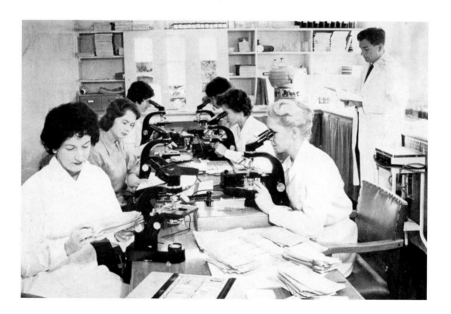

New Zealand's first cytology laboratory, the Cornwall Hospital Obstetric and Gynaecological Unit, 1954. Dr John Sullivan in background.

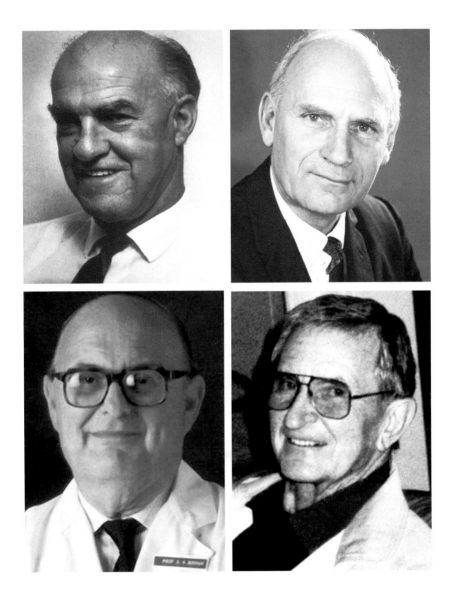

Clockwise from top left: Associate Professor Herbert Green, Dr William (Bill) McIndoe, Dr Malcolm (Jock) McLean, Professor Dennis Bonham.

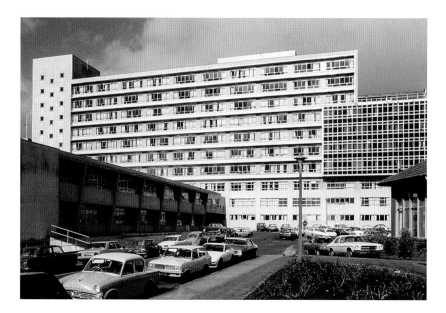

National Women's Hospital in 1973.

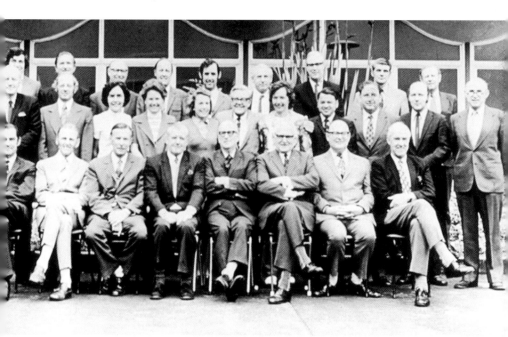

Senior medical staff at National Women's Hospital, 1973. *Front row from left*:
B. Kyle, H. Jameson, B. Faris, B. Grieve, A. Warren, A. Macfarlane,
D. Bonham, H. Green.

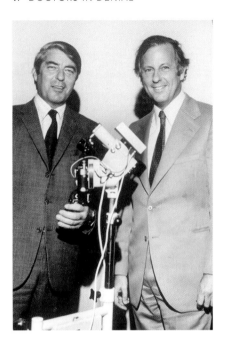

Dr Ellis Pixley and Dr (later Professor) Malcolm Coppleson with a colposcope, about 1975.

Opposite: This figure illustrates that 1.5 per cent of women with normal followup smears (group one) had developed invasive cancer by 20 years; among those women with abnormal followup smears (group two), 18 per cent had developed invasive cancer by 10 years and 36 per cent had developed cancer by 20 years. (McIndoe, McLean, Jones & Mullins, reprinted from *Obstetrics & Gynecology* 64, 1984, 451–58)

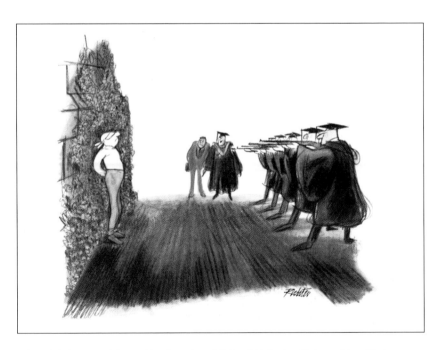

'It's publish or perish, and he hasn't published.' Mischa Richter, *New Yorker*, 28 May 1966. Green didn't want to be left behind Liley and Liggins on the academic tree.

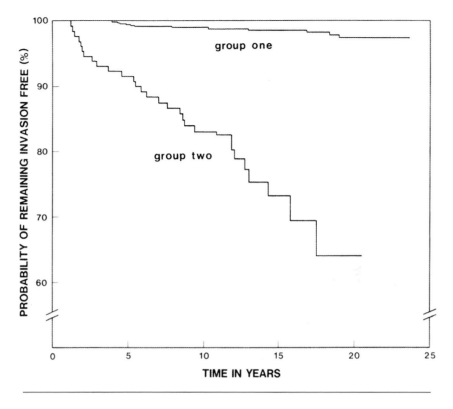

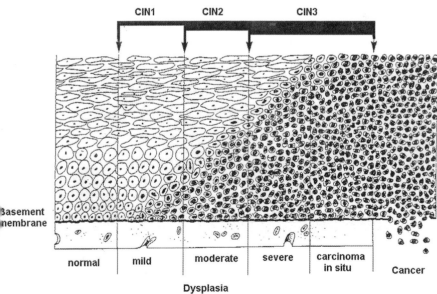

This diagram shows the progression of cellular abnormalities from a normal cervix through carcinoma *in-situ* (CIS) to invasive cancer.

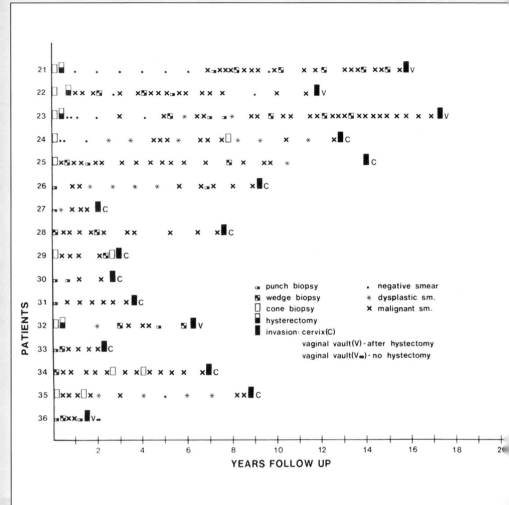

A figure from the 1984 paper showing the disease progression in 16 women who developed invasive cervical cancer. Note the many years of major smear abnormalities and the absence of any definitive treatment of cervix or vaginal CIS. (McIndoe, McLean, Jones & Mullins, reprinted from *Obstetrics & Gynecology* 64, 1984, 451–58.)

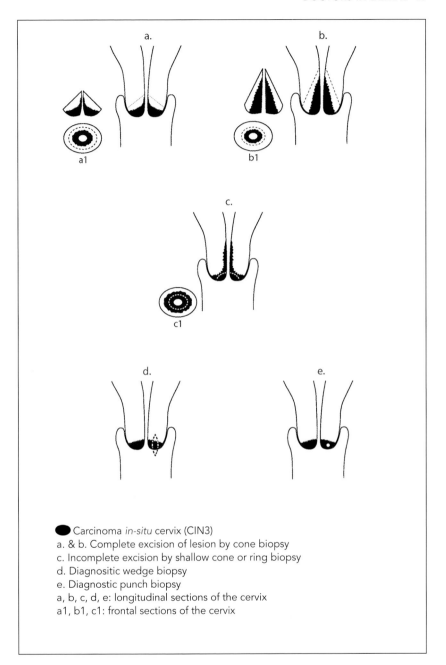

● Carcinoma *in-situ* cervix (CIN3)
a. & b. Complete excision of lesion by cone biopsy
c. Incomplete excision by shallow cone or ring biopsy
d. Diagnositic wedge biopsy
e. Diagnostic punch biopsy
a, b, c, d, e: longitudinal sections of the cervix
a1, b1, c1: frontal sections of the cervix

Different types of cervical biopsy and their effect on the excision of CIS.

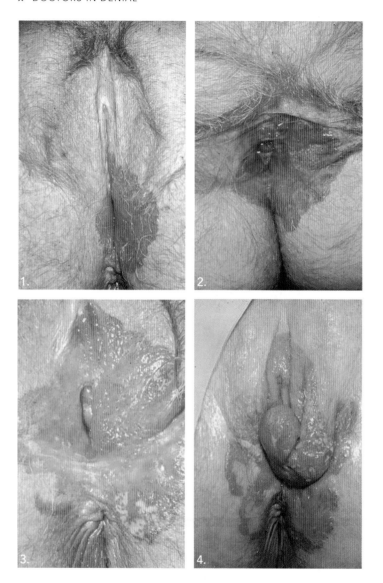

Phoebe's vulva, illustrating the progression of untreated vulval CIS to invasive cancers. *Clockwise from top left*: **1**. November 1970: Green took a small diagnostic biopsy that showed CIS of the vulva, but did not treat it. At that time, removal would have been a simple operation. **2**. In April 1972 Phoebe had two biopsies taken, both reported as vulval CIS. **3**. In January 1975 biopsies from three sites all reported invasive cancer, but Green wrote, 'I do not agree with the diagnosis of squamous carcinoma.' **4**. In September 1976 the operative specimen revealed four separate invasive carcinomas of the vulva arising in an 'actively progressing field of carcinoma *in-situ*'.

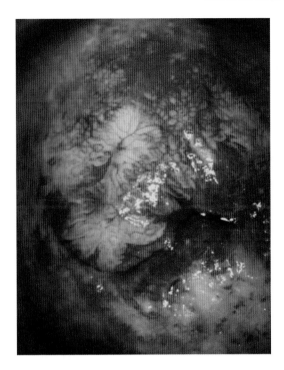

A colposcopy photograph of a cervix with an extensive area of grossly abnormal blood vessels. This is similar to what Green would have seen in many longstanding cases of CIS (CIN 3). The possibility of early invasive cervical cancer can only be excluded by biopsy. (Photo courtesy of Michael Campion.)

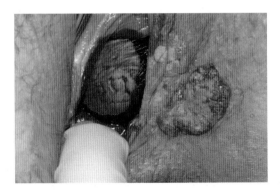

In this photograph of a lower anterior vagina and adjacent vulva, normal vaginal skin has been stained dark brown and the paler vaginal skin is CIS. The flattish pink and white skin on the vulva is CIS and merges into to a small, raised, cancerous tumour.

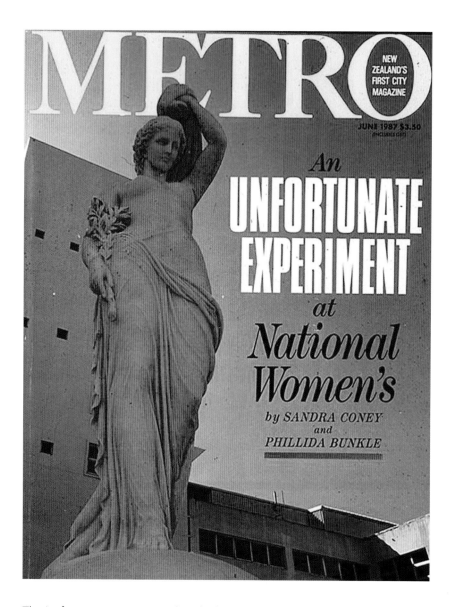

The 'unfortunate experiment' hits the headlines. *Metro*, June 1987.

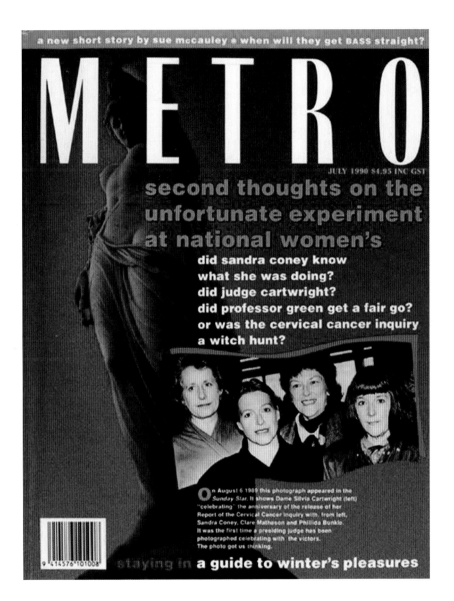

The beginning of revisionism: 'Second thoughts', *Metro*, July 1990.

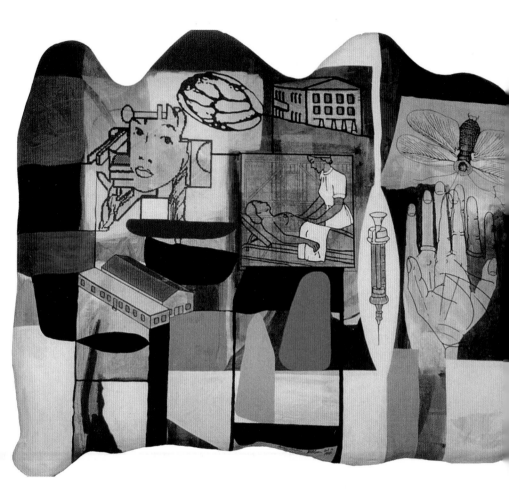

Battery Chickens, a work influenced by the 'unfortunate experiment',
by Richard Killeen, 1988. (Acrylic and collage on polystyrene. From the Christopher Marshall
Collection, reproduced with the permission of the artist.)

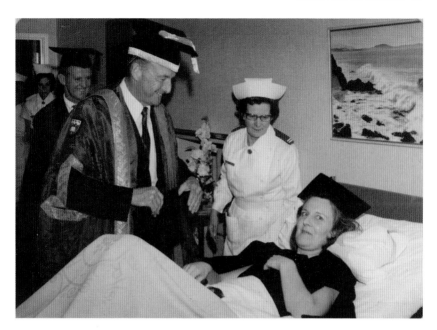

Justice Graham Speight, Chancellor of the University of Auckland, 'capping' a patient in Green's ward, with Sister Fisher in support, c.1975.

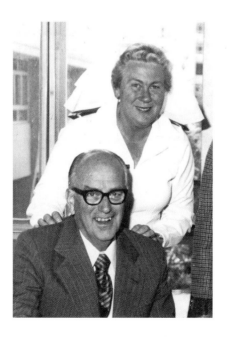

Matron Verna Murray with medical superintendent Dr Algar Warren, 1977.

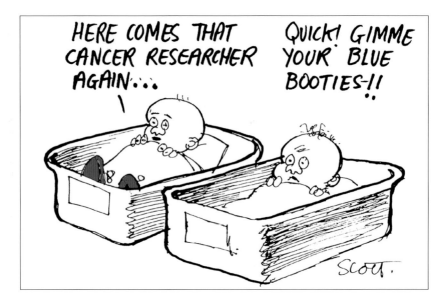

Tom Scott's cartoon illustrating the 'baby smear' episode. Tom Scott, *Evening Post*, 12 November 1987. (Reproduced with the kind permission of the artist.)

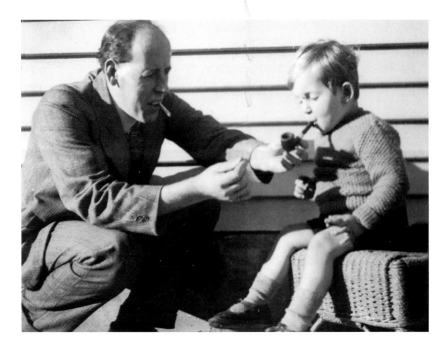

Yesterday's actions should not necessarily be judged by today's standards. The author receives instruction from his father.

lawyer, in the High Court, unsuccessfully attempted to have the key issue of whether there was a failure adequately to treat carcinoma *in-situ* (CIS) at NWH removed from the terms of reference of the inquiry.[31]

Like Green's, Bonham's responses to questions tended to be vague and convoluted. Despite being the professor in charge of the Postgraduate School of Obstetrics and Gynaecology, and chairman of both the Hospital Medical Committee and the Ethics Committee, he was either too 'junior', 'learning', 'didn't remember', 'wasn't told' or was 'not responsible'. Wherever possible, by innuendo or by direct comment about 'colposcopic miss[es]', he blamed McIndoe. Although he did not consider himself an expert, he said he had worked in the field of cancer prevention for a number of years in England and was 'well aware of the debate about the nature of carcinoma *in-situ* … with a 10% [progression] figure, but I am prepared to take it down to 5% and up to 30%'. He did not agree with Green's earlier concession that 'the 1966 policy was, in a strict medical sense, a research programme into the natural history of carcinoma *in-situ*', although there was an information 'spin-off'.[32] Green and Bonham were by now at or near the end of their careers. Used to power and status in their internationally rated department, they equivocated and obfuscated, shifting the blame and refusing to acccept responsibility.

Bonham said it was 'absolute nonsense' that his correspondence with Bunkle and her employer, Victoria University of Wellington, and the NWH medical superintendent regarding our then forthcoming paper was designed 'to throw those people who were looking into the issue off the scent'. When questioned about the paper he said it was published in a 'second line' journal, it was difficult to read, there was no formal discussion about it at the hospital, and he could not recall my giving him a prepublication copy, although he admitted he had read it. Green never submitted prepublication copies of his papers to Bonham, but the latter thought we should have discussed our 1984 paper 'with someone on our side of the hospital'. 'They were', he said, 'unethically describing Green's cases to some extent and poking the finger a bit at him. There are innuendoes in the paper that shouldn't be there.'[33]

Following lengthy cross-examination Bonham finally conceded that he was unable to challenge either the paper's methodology or its conclusions, and that his first formal response to it was at the inquiry. He declined to define the word 'research', saying it was not possible, and since Green's proposal was not a trial there was no need for comment. Later he said 'it was what every doctor did with every patient all the time'. He also said that by 1984 he 'saw little need to review the method of managing [carcinoma *in-situ*]' because he believed 'Green was performing cone biopsies [before his retirement] and the remainder of the staff were treating their own patients'. He could not say the women were not being treated because they constantly had biopsies and Green was 'continually searching for invasive cancer'. Bonham was not concerned about the programme because Green's 'results seemed to prove his point' – although he had wondered if they were 'too good to be true'. When McIndoe and McLean had complained, Bonham was surprised. He considered that, rather than McIndoe criticising Green, he, as the colposcopist, 'should have been looking a little inwardly'. The Macfarlane report 'did not indicate ... urgent clinical action or changes were needed' and, Bonham said euphemistically, the patients' 'problems had been resolved – their problems had settled'.[34]

I believe Bonham's memories of the role of the Hospital Medical Committee in relation to its ethical duties were probably a fair reflection of the views of doctors of the time. He believed it 'had certain ethical responsibilities', but did not believe that 'we regarded ourselves as an ethical committee'. He added, 'I was learning about matters of ethics at that time.' Bonham finished his cross-examination with an unusual observation: 'I have on a number of occasions in recent years found Dr Green does not immediately perceive the true point of the question you are asking him.'[35]

Despite Tony Baird's strong, confident public support for Green, Bonham and the hospital, his performance in the witness box as chairman of the New Zealand Medical Association was uncertain, diffident and defensive. He had had a specialist qualification for 14 years, had worked for Green in the mid-1970s and been a locum medical superintendent, and yet claimed no knowledge of the criticisms then being expressed in the hospital about Green's study. He pleaded ignorance; he was 'learning'; he was unaware 'there was a different school of thought', finding out about it for the first time in the *Metro* article; he stated that 'there is considerable doubt whether there is progression of carcinoma *in-situ* to invasive cancer'; and he was 'unaware of anything else going on [in the hospital] that is not orthodox or standard', or of Green's iconoclastic views. He further suggested that 'doing nothing is a form of treatment'.[36]

Bruce Faris also defended Green, denying there was a trial, emphasising that 'clinical freedom' was 'jealously guarded' by doctors all around the world and was 'an absolute necessity'. He said he had not reviewed any of the 15 (of 29) cases that had been excluded from the working party report in 1975.[37]

Green was able to muster only three overseas supporters to assist in his defence, and in the end they were of no real assistance. Dr Ellis Pixley, from Perth, Green's old colleague in the fetal cervix research in the 1960s, agreed to come as a witness but was not adequately briefed; for example, he had not been shown a copy of the 1966 proposal. I knew Pixley fairly well. On arriving in Auckland he phoned me and asked, 'What is all this about?' When I told him some of the background to the inquiry his response was a colourful expletive. In the witness stand he brought both colour and character and followed his own dictum: 'Improper prior preparation makes piss poor presentation.'[38] His responses were conventional and truthful. He disagreed with Green's management and said he had 'expressed some concerns about what was going on' during his visits to NWH in 1967 and 1974. He had heard me present our 1984 paper in Tokyo and agreed with our conclusions. In the end he provided no support for Green.[39]

Two Japanese doctors, both involved in the prevention of cervical cancer by screening, diagnosis and the treatment of precursor lesions, were placed in the invidious position of supporting Green despite using conventional treatment in their home country. Green had invited both men, Sadamu Noda and Minoru Ueki, to work at NWH, and I had subsequently worked with both of them. They followed the Japanese custom of showing respect, gratitude and loyalty to an old teacher, mentor and friend. In Japanese fashion the younger doctor, Ueki, deferred to his senior colleague throughout their evidence. Their comments backed Green but their responses were hampered by the limitations of their command of English. They were not prepared to criticise Green, but in the end neither provided any substantial support for him either.[40]

During the course of the inquiry there were suggestions from the Hospital Board lawyer, David Morris, that NWH would defend the allegations of inadequate treatment of CIS by reviewing all cases in the hospital. One would assume this review would be performed independently – if the administrators had learned anything from the experience of the working party. Instead Honeyman and Collison invited Drs Murray Jamieson and Andrew Mackintosh to do the review as 'clinical witnesses', since they 'knew what to look for and where to find it'. Former students of Green, neither performed preinvasive or colposcopy work in the hospital and they were now his replacements on D (cervix cancer) Team. Although the inquiry focused on cases managed up to 1976, Jamieson and Mackintosh declined 'to provide opinions regarding adequacy of treatment' before this time because of their 'inexperience'.[41] At the inquiry I described their almost incomprehensible 46-page summary as being like a 'London bus timetable'. In a number of cases included in our 1984 paper they followed Green's practice of reclassifying them as 'invasion at the outset' – a possibility, given the inadequacy of many of Green's biopsies. Later Cartwright reported that her medical advisers 'were unable to accept [their figures] as accurate in all cases'.[42]

Standing back, I found it easy to discern a clash between the old, patriarchal medical culture and the new, forceful, questioning feminist culture, but the old NWH establishment did not see this.

* * *

Judge Cartwright referred to the visiting international authorities as the 'high priests' in the field and clearly welcomed and respected their independent opinions.[43] Professors Per Kolstad from Oslo, Ralph Richart from New York, Malcolm Coppleson from Sydney, Drs Joe Jordan from Birmingham, Colin Laverty from Sydney and Ellis Pixley from Perth were all familiar with the historical background relating to the natural history of CIS of the cervix, its management internationally, and with Green's 'atypical viewpoint' as set out in his published papers.

Richart had only a limited time in New Zealand and his evidence was interpolated between Green's evidence. Before Richart's appearance Green had made small progress, drawing attention to a number of inconsequential errors in the *Metro* article. The introduction of Richart into the witness box changed everything. Green's ambiguity was replaced by Richart's clarity of thought and presentation – from the overwhelming evidence of the long-established basis for the precancerous nature of CIS, to the roles of cytology, histology and colposcopy in diagnosis, and the importance of adequate treatment. Richart said, 'I have known of no one except Dr Green who would recommend prospectively following patients with persistent carcinoma *in-situ* of the cervix, vulva or vagina rather than treating them and eradicating the lesion.'[44]

Joe Jordan, an internationally respected clinician-colposcopist, had vivid memories of Green's visit to Birmingham in 1971 and the debate accompanied by 'violent confrontation and disagreement' with Professor Hugh McLaren, Britain's most powerful advocate for cervical screening.[45] He believed Green's experiment should never have been allowed to begin in the first place: 'From 1966 onwards I know of no unit other than Professor Green's which was prepared to allow patients with carcinoma *in-situ* to continue without [definitive] treatment.' Following a review of the case notes of women with extensive longstanding CIS, Jordan was forced to admit that Green was ultimately faced with a management 'dilemma'. But these cases became a dilemma only as a consequence of the more than two decades of neglect. He was adamant all women with CIS should be treated with the aim of eradicating the disease.[46]

Professor Per Kolstad's appearance in the witness stand gave me a sense of déjà vu. His words mirrored those he had spoken to Green, McIndoe and me in 1973; the only difference was that 14 years later they were being considered by a judge. He described a case he had reviewed in 1973 as 'an example of mismanagement that should never have occurred', another as 'severe mismanagement' and yet another as 'terrifying mismanagement'. He also observed he was 'really horrified about the attitude of Dr Green'.[47]

The commission, believing Coppleson's evidence was crucial, interviewed him in Sydney. He stressed that, in the 1960s, Green was one of the few gynaecologists to endorse a conservative, non-hysterectomy, cone biopsy approach to treatment. Coppleson said that irrespective of any particular conservative technique, total eradication of CIS and normal follow-up smears were mandatory. He 'wonder[ed] how [Green's] trial reached the disaster phase … assum[ing] Green's authority continued to prevail' over McIndoe and McLean's concerns.[48]

Professor David Skegg was New Zealand's most erudite witness. He stressed that all the evidence, including Green's own publications, pointed to the experimental nature of the research. Skegg noted that the only criticisms he had received of his own 1985 paper, designed to promote and improve a more effective cervical screening programme in New Zealand, had come from the academic unit at NWH.[49] Bonham had stressed to Skegg: 'You will be receiving fairly critical suggestions from a number of my colleagues.' Murray Jamieson, head of the cervical cancer team, said he 'did not accept there is any compelling evidence [that] cytological screening is an effective preventive measure … every day in my clinical teaching I fight the good fight *against tests*, and for the *history and examination* [Jamieson's emphases].[50] As all doctors and many women know, Pap screening programmes are designed to detect microscopic abnormalities in asymptomatic women with clinically normal cervices and the test is *less* reliable when cancer is present because of the necrotic material and inflammation.

The low point in the inquiry (and the high point for the media) was the unexpected revelation by Michael Churchouse that between 1963 and 1966, on Green's instruction, nurses had taken 2200 vaginal smears from newborn girls without the knowledge or consent of their mothers.[51] As described in Chapter 2, Green considered the possibility that abnormal-looking but harmless cells would, on occasion, be detected in these infants, confirming his view of the innocent nature of CIS. Tony Baird leapt to Green's defence, saying 'at most 150 smears were taken from newborn babies and these were "coincidentally" during routine checks [i.e. swabs] for infections such as staphylococcus and gonorrhoea'.[52] Professor Colin Mantell stirred things up when he stated on television that vaginal swabs were currently being taken from babies at Middlemore Hospital when there was a question of infection. His paediatric colleagues disputed his assertion and he was forced to retract these comments. This misplaced loyalty rebounded when Churchouse's statement that 2200 'smears' (and *not* swabs) were taken was confirmed. He said 'the smears taken by cotton-tipped applicators were fixed and suitable for cytological examination for abnormal cells, but not suitable for bacterial examination'.[53]

* * *

The stress I experienced as a witness at the inquiry was increased immeasurably by my position as a whistle-blower. My attempt to give some credit to Green and his loyal secretary, Miss Owen, for their diligence in following up women, was misinterpreted as my giving credit to Green's experiment. Coney, in her book, accused me of being placatory. Had she known of my personal turmoil she might have been more generous. My friend, mentor and supporter, McIndoe, was dead; my wife, Barbara, was likely to die; I had a young family about to be motherless; and I was persona non grata among my colleagues. At least in the short term I needed to remain working at NWH, and my loyalty to my hospital and patients remained unchanged. How could I, on a public stage, in front of television cameras and the baying press, condemn my colleagues? It would have been professional suicide. Coney was correct – I was placatory.

To Coney's lawyer, Rodney Harrison, I explained why I had accepted McIndoe and McLean's suggestion that I assist them in writing the paper: 'Quite simply this material was in my view the most important modern evidence which substantiated the earlier view regarding the invasive potential of the precursor lesions (carcinoma *in-situ*).' I pointed out that several papers on the subject had already been published from the NWH, 'some indicating carcinoma *in-situ* of the cervix had a relatively unimportant invasive potential and others which doubted the value of mass cervical cytology screening'. I therefore believed 'it would have been morally wrong not to publish the material in a major international journal. Although the results presented in our 1984 paper have come under microscopic examination during this Inquiry they state nothing more than the views held by the rest of the gynaecologists in this country and overseas.'

I concluded my evidence by describing the 'immense impact' of the inquiry on everyone working at NWH. 'Differences of opinion have been exaggerated, creating an atmosphere of suspicion and mistrust. Some of the issues being examined ... would under normal circumstances have been regarded as variations in clinical opinions.'

Anyone who has worked in a large institution is all too familiar with the effects of personality differences and the manoeuvring for positions of power and influence. It is important in medical practice such differences be subjugated and the best interests of the patients become the prime concern. Those of us involved in this Inquiry have had to face the ... choice between loyalty to longstanding and trusted colleagues and to the profession, and to the best interests of our patients ... Looked at objectively the decision between these alternatives seems easy, but for those of us emotionally involved the issues have become blurred.

The commission had set me a number of tasks – evidence to gather to present to the inquiry. First, what was the outcome in women presenting with CIS in the three years immediately following the cut-off date for women included in our 1984 paper? Were they receiving adequate treatment at the time? My enquiries showed that only three (0.75 per cent) of 426 women had developed cancer during those three years – a figure consistent with other published series of treated CIS.[54] This was good news, clear evidence that current patients were being managed appropriately. The backlog of Green's inadequately treated cases would emerge later.

Second, the earliest stage of cervical cancer is termed microinvasion. Here small groups of cells from the deepest layer of CIS invade through the basement membrane of the epithelial surface, creating a microscopic cancer. The deeper the cells penetrate, the greater the risk the cells will spread beyond the cervix, potentially threatening the woman's life. Although Green was never given permission to study women with microinvasion, he made a personal decision to include them in his study of CIS, believing they were part of the same condition. This illustrates perfectly Green's confused logic: on the one hand he said CIS and invasive cancer were separate conditions, yet in this context he believed CIS with microscopic invasive cancer was part of the same condition. The microscopic progression of CIS cells to microinvasion provides one of the important pieces of evidence that CIS and invasive cancer are linked. I examined the outcome in 110 of these women: most had received adequate treatment. However, 11 of 23 women (48 per cent) with continuing smear abnormalities following inadequate treatment developed higher-stage cancers.[55]

Third, the commission was naturally interested in the outcome of 75 women who had 'shown evidence of persistent disease [CIS] after various initial treatments', reported by Green in 1970. At the time of the inquiry 14 (19 per cent) of the women had developed cancer. At the time of a subsequent review in 2007, 25 (33 per cent) had developed cancer.[56]

At the end of the inquiry none of the expert witnesses was able to sustain Green's hypothesis that 'the patient with in-situ cancer has only the normal [future] chance of developing invasive cancer'.[57]

* * *

Academic freedom is jealously guarded by university employees: the role of the university as critic and conscience of a society is now guaranteed by the Education Act 1989. Margaret Vennell, a senior lecturer in the Auckland University Law School, was called by Judge Cartwright as an expert witness at the inquiry in the area of informed consent, and she gave evidence to the inquiry in a private capacity.[58] Counsel for the university publicly dissociated the institution from her evidence 'in order that the university's interests be protected'.

Extraordinarily, Warwick Nicoll, the university registrar, afterwards 'reprimanded' Margaret Vennell and 'accused [her] of disloyalty to the university by reason of [her] giving evidence as a witness at the Inquiry'.[59] She wrote to Nicoll explaining her actions and he responded with a begrudging apology. Vennell described being subjected subsequently to a departmental 'trial' by her dean, Jock Brookfield, who acted as the prosecutor, expressing 'concerns' about her actions and asking her why she had not informed him, as head of department, of her intention to give evidence, since the university was involved and represented in the inquiry.[60]

Counsel for three other parties at the inquiry brought this matter to the attention of Judge Cartwright, who undertook to interview Vennell. Silvia Cartwright wrote a strongly worded letter to the chancellor expressing her disquiet. She said a witness called by a commission 'ought not have her personal motives queried'; university employees should be 'reassured that the concept of academic freedom will be honoured'; and 'the content of the evidence ought not to be the subject of criticism or comment by the employer'.[61] This sad episode created longstanding bitterness between Margaret Vennell and the University of Auckland.

* * *

A number of women's groups made brief appearances towards the end of the inquiry. Their principal concerns were patients, professionals and power. Patients need to be treated with respect as equals; the medical profession, having been accountable only to itself, needed to change its ways.

Mary O'Regan, secretary to the Ministry of Women's Affairs, stressed the centrality to the inquiry of 'the very basic issue of the relationship between the medical profession as "experts" and women as consumers of health services. The dynamic is one of power versus powerlessness.' She noted the irony that the very nature of the inquiry had 'mirrored this dynamic'.

There have been days spent listening to medical experts. A great deal of money has been spent on bringing their expertise and perspective to this Inquiry. But women have not had access to comparable facilities to ensure … their voices are heard. Women all over the country have been outraged by what they have been hearing, especially as they have identified with the powerlessness of the women who entrusted the medical experts with their bodies and their lives …

Women must never again be used as unknowing subjects in research projects such as that which is the subject for this Inquiry. When we go to get treatment for a medical condition we must be given the best treatment possible and know what is being done to us. No information or treatment should be withheld from us in order to test a doctor's hypothesis. This is a gross breach of the faith that patients have been socialised to have in their doctors.[62]

From my perspective the message about power was too narrow. The reason for the inquiry was an unethical experiment brought about by the unequal distribution of power in a department of a leading university – a powerful medical hierarchy that knowingly ignored the pleas of the 'little men', McIndoe and McLean, at the end of the chain. It could have been a power imbalance in any institution.

The Auckland Hospital Board and the university offered almost no defence of the actions of their academic clinical staff at NWH. It became increasingly evident that because so many patients were harmed by Green's seriously flawed study, no real defence could be offered. None-too-subtle attempts to denigrate us, the authors of the 1984 and 1986 papers, failed, and although we were naturally anxious about what the Cartwright Report might say, we were very relieved when it was published on 5 August 1988.

'I have come to believe,' Cartwright wrote, 'Doctor Green was trying to prove a personal belief. The inference that carcinoma *in-situ* will progress to invasive cancer in only a very small proportion of cases is incorrect. It was an attempt to prove a theory [that] lacked scientific validity and little attention was given to ethical considerations.' There was, she considered, 'no serious suggestion that he … had anything but a benevolent attitude to his patients'. The senior medical staff had 'no will to confront and resolve difficult issues … The publication of the 1984 and 1986 papers represented the medical profession's last opportunity to exercise its own assessment. It failed to do so.'

In her view, 'McIndoe and his co-authors and the authors of the *Metro* article shared a similar experience: they met with a wall of resistance particularly from the academic unit at NWH. All the authors used an extraordinary determination to tell the truth. I have the eerie impression that Dr McIndoe's memoranda and notes were almost prophetic.'[63] Judge Cartwright found that the 'criticisms of the McIndoe paper do not stand up to examination.'[64]

The Cartwright Report has had more positive impact on the way doctors practise medicine in New Zealand than any other single event.[65] Understandably, New Zealand doctors have not thanked us for our role. It was a pyrrhic victory.

CHAPTER 10

AFTERMATH

We are not the doctors, we are the disease.

DOUGLAS ROBB

IMMEDIATELY AFTER THE PUBLICATION of the Cartwright Report the response of the medical profession and Green's supporters was relatively muted. Many doctors were shocked by the revelations in the report and their coverage by the media, but few were prepared to voice their opinions publicly. Coney was correct in her observation that 'most doctors had simply gone to ground'.[1]

As chairman of the New Zealand Medical Association and a member of the senior medical staff at NWH, Tony Baird was placed in the invidious position of having to express support publicly for both the findings of the report and the beleaguered medical profession, while holding personal reservations about the inquiry and its findings. He acknowledged 'those who have been hurt by the medical profession ... the anger amongst women's groups ... younger doctors who have all been condemned by the actions of their predecessors ... things are not perfect ... there is a lot to be done and a need to change the behaviour of some medical practitioners'.[2]

At least he made an acknowledgement, but this was not the time 'to change the behaviour' of some unidentified doctors. It was the time to admit that there had been an unethical experiment in his hospital, and many women and their families had suffered. It was the time to apologise profusely. At a meeting of the Hospital Medical Committee on 18 August 1988, 10 days after the release of the Cartwright Report, Gabrielle Collison noted that there had been no formal record of the cessation of Green's study. The committee duly confirmed that 'the 1966 trial has ceased'.[3] The findings of the inquiry were not even discussed.

At the next meeting of the committee, on 15 September 1988, Dr Barry Lowe and I moved that the following statement be released: 'The senior medical staff of the National Women's Hospital express their regret and sympathy to the patients and their families [whom] Judge Cartwright described in the Report as "a minority of women" whose management resulted in persistent disease, the development of invasive cancer and in some cases death.'[4] The motion was carried unanimously.

An urgent meeting was called a week later. Collison reported that some members of the senior medical staff had lobbied her and requested further discussion of the statement, so she reopened the matter. On this occasion no consensus was reached, and it was resolved that 'no public statement should be issued on behalf of the Hospital Medical Committee at this time'.[5] Clearly, attitudes of the majority of the senior medical staff had not changed since the inquiry report. Professor Colin Mantell tabled a letter suggesting a series of 'special meetings' be set up to consider the recommendations of the Cartwright Report. Baird supported the suggestion, but added a rider: 'Mr Jones, Dr McLean and Mr Churchouse be asked to provide their own reports.'[6] Obviously, the opinions of the whistle-blowers were not perceived as likely to fit with the views of the committee's general membership.

The attitude of the Royal New Zealand College of Obstetricians and Gynaecologists (RNZCOG) was even more remarkable. This was the nationwide body with responsibility for standards within the specialty. The college hierarchy was initially reluctant to call a special meeting to discuss the Cartwright Report. However, a threat by some younger Wellington fellows to invoke the articles of association prompted action, and the president, Professor Dick Seddon, called an extraordinary general meeting in Wellington on 23 September 1988.[7] Fifty fellows attended and apologies were received from 45.

I approached the meeting with considerable trepidation. McIndoe was dead and I had to represent him as well as myself. I made an extempore presentation of the background to, and the reasons for, writing the 1984 paper. Ian Ronayne, previously a covert supporter, decided to demonstrate publicly his support for us and read a prepared address to the meeting. He began by noting that he was 'the only one here today who was present at the hospital throughout the period investigated'. He described the Cartwright Report as 'a full account, [a] well documented and factually correct summary [that] must be accepted as such. We must learn from the past faults of the academic unit at NWH and those members of D team [who] were knowledgeably involved. The procedures allowed to be followed by these consultants must not be allowed to occur again and greater control over experimental procedures must be witnessed.' When overseas, he 'had to be defensive when they knew I was from N.W.H. and I was confronted with remarks such as "Is Green still at it?"' When Ronayne expressed his concern to Dr Liam Wright, he was told, 'Don't rock the boat; I have to work with him.'[8]

Ronayne also rebutted Baird's opinion that 'the McIndoe et al paper was a personal vindictive attack on the academic and associated D team members'. It was, he said, 'my pleasure to be associated with the late Bill McIndoe in the same clinic all his working life and thus I was able to closely observe the profound disquiet he had about Professor Green's policies. This had a long-term effect on his health. The great effort Bill took to ensure total accuracy of his reported data had to be seen to be believed.' He also noted that his own family 'were personally aggrieved to find one of our daughters had a vaginal smear taken 5 days after her delivery. We felt we had been deceived.'[9]

Ronayne concluded:

Many of us have been bracketed with those of our colleagues whose actions have brought us into intense public disrepute. Even now some members of the N.W.H. are not prepared to accept the Inquiry findings.

I believe a press statement should be made by our College after this meeting expressing our public regret for this sorry episode in our history and to reassure the public of our intention to regulate our attitude so this unfortunate experiment will not occur again.

He then proposed a motion that 'Doctors McIndoe, McLean and Jones were morally and scientifically justified in publishing their 1984 and 1986 papers in *Obstetrics and Gynecology*'.[10] Seconded by Mantell, the motion was passed unanimously.

Subsequently, Baird, who had not attended the meeting, wrote to chairman Seddon:

I take exception to the use of the word 'morally' in the motion proposed by Ian Ronayne ... and I wish to formally disassociate myself from the motion. To me it is humbug.

There was a moral duty in all this business, and it involved the care of the women shown by the authors of the '1984 paper' to have been treated inadequately. They had a duty to inform the rest of the staff at National Women's Hospital about what they had found; probably the College as well and more importantly to ensure that the women were looked after. Instead they publish a paper in a journal overseas that very few people in New Zealand read regularly and then do nothing more.

To wait for journalists to show concern for the subjects of the so-called trial is anything but moral in my view and it could be a dereliction of care which, of course, is most unethical. None of this provides any grounds for us to feel self-righteousness or for satisfaction and self-congratulation and I include the authors of the '1984 paper' in that statement.

I wish to give notice of a motion for the Next Annual General Meeting as follows, 'that the word "moral" [sic] be deleted from Mr Ronayne's motion passed at the extraordinary general meeting on Friday 23rd September 1988.[11]

Ronayne stoutly defended his motion at the next meeting and no change was made to it.[12] Baird did not attend either meeting.

Baird's judgement on morality is ironic. We knew he had read our paper, and then told Sandra Coney it was 'wrong', but had done nothing about it for more than two years before he wrote this letter.[13]

At the same meeting on 23 September Dr Gerald Duff proposed the motion: 'That the College express regret and sympathy for the women involved and abhorrence of the events reported in the Inquiry'. That motion was lost. Mantell said the reasons for the lack of response to the report by the postgraduate school 'related largely to the legal implications of such statements and the difficulties in getting media interest'. A motion was then passed: 'That a letter be sent to Professors Green and Bonham expressing hope for them and their families' wellbeing'.[14]

The medical staff of Greenlane Hospital, the immediate neighbour of NWH, arranged a combined meeting of the medical staff of the two hospitals. Some Greenlane doctors were 'concerned about the accusations and allegations in the *New Zealand Medical Journal* and in *Metro*. No longer is it acceptable to lie [down].'[15] It was decided a statement should be made, and 'no longer should flagrantly false accusations be allowed to be made in public without response'.[16]

In September 1988 Dr Roger Hilliker, president of the New Zealand Medical Association, asked the New Zealand Medical Council 'to investigate the conduct of Associate Professor Herbert Green and Professor Dennis Bonham and any other doctor who might have been involved in the affair'.[17] There must have been considerable debate – even possible reluctance to act – within the Medical Council, because it was not until February 1990 that it announced Bonham and Green would face charges of disgraceful conduct in a professional respect, and Bruce Faris and Dick Seddon lesser charges of professional misconduct. The charges against Green did not proceed to a hearing on account of his ill-health. Bonham was found guilty of disgraceful conduct but remained a registered practitioner. Most of the charges against Faris and Seddon were struck out by the High Court in 1992, and on the remainder, in July 1995, each was found guilty of conduct unbecoming a medical practitioner.

The Auckland Women's Health Council expressed concern about the private nature of the hearings and the composition of the 'medically dominated' committees involved. It also suggested other doctors were culpable, particularly those who worked with Green and who must surely have been aware that some of his patients had developed cancer.[18]

* * *

We, the 'whistle-blowers', were not debriefed following the inquiry. We were subjected by senior hospital management and some senior colleagues to the well-recognised pattern of deny, delay, divide and discredit. We received no thanks, no apology.

I have particular disdain for the three medical superintendents-in-chief who chose not to become involved. McLean's wife, Ailsa, had gone directly to Wilton Henley and begged him to intervene – he promised he would but failed to do so. Warren, McIndoe and McLean had pleaded with Fred Moody to do something but he had washed his hands of the issue by saying, 'I delegated my responsibility to thoroughly responsible and trustworthy superintendents and it was their job to do it, not mine.' Leslie Honeyman had undertaken to investigate, following a letter of concern relating to the findings of our 1984 paper, but had done nothing. The medical superintendents at NWH also failed to address the situation. Algar Warren supported McIndoe, McLean and me, but, like the rest of us, was largely dominated by Bonham and Green; Ian Hutchison was ineffective; Gabrielle Collison sided with the hospital establishment. The most senior clinicians were too close, too loyal or too weak to tackle Bonham and Green.

We had not considered going to the media; doctors of our generation did not do that sort of thing. It had taken two media-savvy women to finally bring about action. Sandra Coney, who called herself a moderate feminist, could present a severe persona and was not afraid to question the exalted status of doctors. In 1984 she had noted that feminism was 'increasingly failing to talk to women about their day to day problems, about their work, jobs and childcare'. She sought what she described as 'high-powered, effective, streamlined action'.[19] Along with Phillida Bunkle, she had achieved exactly that in their *Metro* article and the subsequent inquiry.

Our professional organisations were of no assistance. The RNZCOG played an ambiguous role, as did the New Zealand Medical Association. The divisions between the NZMA executive and its chairman, Tony Baird, became evident with the publication, in the association's newsletter of January 1989, of a draft paper by a working party set up to study the implementation of the recommendations contained in the report of the inquiry:

> *Noting ... there is considerable anger amongst the profession that the 1966 trial was allowed to occur, Dr Arthur [chairman of the working party] said it is regrettable ... the trial deteriorated scientifically and ethically and did not change as scientific knowledge advanced, or as adverse results were observed. Dr Arthur says ... it is inexcusable and deplorable that all patients involved did not know they were part of a trial, and that it took a magazine article to bring about an investigation.*[20]

This strongly worded statement had clearly escaped Baird's scrutiny, because in the next issue he made the following retraction: 'The January [NZMA] newsletter contained an item entitled "Cartwright Report" which was printed in error ... The statement does not represent NZMA policy and its inclusion in the Newsletter is regretted.'[21] A similar gulf was apparent from the minutes of an earlier (August 1988) council meeting, which endorsed the assertion that the modes of treatment undertaken at NWH from 1966 were 'patently unethical'.[22]

Writing in the *New Zealand Listener* in September 1988, Sandra Coney admitted to being cynical about the numerous university, hospital and hospital board working parties 'where doctors and others go through the motion of instituting reform, while actually doing very little'. 'Left to themselves,' she observed, *the doctors will not get it right, due to a persistent inability to see their patients as equals ... I suspect the inertia and resistance of the system will be the biggest obstacles to change. No one likes to relinquish power, least of all Dr God. Unless women and other community groups insert themselves into the process of reform rather forcibly, then, in the judge's words, 'the kind of events disclosed during this Inquiry may well occur again'.*[23]

A correspondent to the *Listener* asked why there had been no apology from the dean of medicine, and pointed to the 'failure of the University to seek the truth, or apologise to McIndoe, McLean, and Jones who had exposed the scandal'.[24]

* * *

On 12 March 1989, nine months after the Cartwright Inquiry finished, a headline in the *Dominion Sunday Times* proclaimed: 'Cartwright Report based on a scam'.[25] Dr Graeme Overton, an obstetrician and gynaecologist at NWH had reanalysed the 1984 paper and the *Metro* article and claimed that the Cartwright Report was 'based on a false interpretation of the figures'. It was Overton who had diagnosed Clare Matheson's ('Ruth's') cancer and told her she had been left sitting on a 'time bomb'. Now, extraordinarily, he did an about-face, claiming that the Cartwright Inquiry (and Coney and Bunkle) had misinterpreted the statistics in the 1984 paper and that the case against Green's experiment was not proven.

As I would tell journalist Carroll du Chateau many years later, Overton and his colleagues failed to grasp that, while many of Green's patients were eventually partially treated, their treatment was totally inadequate, the disease persisted and the women remained at risk of cancer. Nevertheless, at its next meeting, the Auckland Division of Obstetrics and Gynaecology unanimously voted its support for Overton's reinterpretation.[26] At this point it seemed to me there was a campaign by a group of gynaecologists to discredit the findings of the inquiry. In my view they were not interested in bringing about change, only fighting it.

Metro magazine then did its own about-face by publishing, in July 1990, Jan Corbett's 'Second thoughts on the unfortunate experiment', based largely on Overton's analysis.[27] My colleagues Murray Jamieson and Andrew Mackintosh from the Auckland Division of Obstetrics and Gynaecology provided public support for this article, describing it as 'a moderate and balanced consideration of the relevant matters'. In their view it raised 'questions regarding the Cartwright Inquiry which demand a better answer than has been provided by official sources to date'. They described the inquiry as 'a carefully orchestrated campaign of discreditation'.[28]

Overton had contacted Peter Mullins, who did the statistics for the 1984 paper. He was quoted in Corbett's article as confessing to 'having his own doubts about some aspects' of the paper and never being happy 'with the classification criteria' used.[29] Mullins, like Overton, had never approached us to discuss his concerns. He was fully aware of the contentious issues raised at the Cartwright Inquiry and could have come forward at the time, but chose to remain silent. Scientific practice behoves an author who subsequently believes the content of a paper to which he or she has contributed to be in error to communicate with his fellow authors and, if necessary, with the journal editor, setting out the issues in question and requesting the publication of a retraction. Thirty years later Mullins has done neither.

In my response to Corbett's article I observed that if we combined all cases into one group, we still ended up with the world's worst figures, with approximately one woman in 20 with CIS developing cancer. I explained that

> our 1984 paper was written because the authors felt a responsibility to ensure the outcome of the 1966 study was analysed and published. Such publication would correct and complete the earlier publications by other authors; inform the medical profession; and also inform hospital authorities. The 1966 study, despite the tragedy of suffering and death, did produce data which would never again be available and which has provided the best published proof that CIS of the cervix can progress to invasive cancer. It confirms the many other papers that say this. There is none that disproves it.

The medical opponents of the paper's conclusions were 'conducting a guerrilla campaign. None had responded in the medical press; nor had they participated in the inquiry or taken court proceedings regarding its findings'.[30]

A heated correspondence in *Metro* followed, including a letter from Baird, this time as chairman of the Auckland Division of Obstetrics and Gynaecology. He not only said that in our paper we had 'misinterpreted' the data, but also alleged that we 'selected' patients, implying that we had manipulated the data.[31]

Dr Erich Geiringer, an iconoclast well known to my fellow students at the Otago Medical School in the 1960s, wrote a stinging article in *Metro* in October 1990 entitled, 'The triumph of victimocracy'. He was highly critical of Cartwright, claiming that her lack of medical knowledge limited her ability to interpret facts and formulate recommendations. He described Green's study as 'a poorly designed experiment fraught with ethical danger', but ultimately, Geiringer saw the inquiry as having been 'ruthlessly exploited by the feminist and official lobby, with the help of the media, to discredit and intimidate the medical profession who largely and characteristically caved in'.[32]

In a strongly worded statement issued in September 1990, Minister of Health Helen Clark had rebutted criticisms of the Cartwright Report. She reiterated our statement that untreated CIS cannot safely be ignored and noted that the figures used in the 'Second thoughts' article relied on Jamieson and Mackintosh's in-house review of CIS at NWH. Cartwright's medical advisers had been 'unable to accept [Jamieson and Mackintosh's figures] as accurate in all cases'.[33]

And in response to Overton's attempt to rewrite history, an *Auckland Star* editorial titled 'Doctor does not know best' described the 'intransigence and arrogance of some sections of the medical profession' that were 'sadly evident' in Overton's move:

> *Every one of the points raised by Dr Overton, particularly the issue of Dr William McIndoe's statistical analysis presented in evidence to the inquiry, were exhaustively analysed by the Cervical Cancer Inquiry.*
>
> *The medical profession generally has had difficulty accepting any creed other than 'doctor knows best' and indifference to the notion of patients' rights. The unfortunate but prevailing medical opinion among a strong group of unenlightened practitioners is that doctors have a monopoly on what's right for patients.*
>
> *Some of these doctors who publicly display disbelief and exhibit defiance are still stalking the corridors of National Women's [Hospital].*[34]

Judge Cartwright's specific comments had been directed at the 'unfortunate experiment', but she had also reflected on the attitudes and conduct of the profession as a whole:

*I reserve particular disquiet not only for the fate of the 30 patients
mentioned in the McIndoe et al paper, to whom there was a special duty
owed, but also for the future of peer review within the medical profession,
if it cannot confront issues squarely and resolve them after such
sustained, detailed and well-documented statements of concern about the
treatment of a group of patients and the minority view advocated by one
clinician.*[35]

One unseemly aspect in the post-Cartwright era was a media stoush
between Baird and Coney over the exact number of women who died as a
result of Green's experiment.[36] The exact number has never been confirmed.
Sandra Coney has documented 30 deaths, but this figure does not include
women like Phoebe (see Chapter Six) with cancer of the vulva, women like
Mabel (see Chapter Twelve) who died overseas, or those who have died
since the inquiry. No woman with diagnosed CIS should die of a CIS-
related cancer.

What was missed of course is the much larger group of New Zealand
women who developed cancer – some of whom died – as a consequence
of Green's opposition to national cervical screening.[37] Associate Professor
Brian Cox, an expert in cancer screening and director of the Hugh Adam
Cancer Epidemiology Unit at the Otago Medical School, has calculated
that if, as George Wied had suggested, a national screening programme
had been introduced in 1959, rather than in 1991, about 3100 women
over those 32 years 'would have had invasive cervical cancer prevented'.
The organised programmes introduced in some Scandinavian countries in
the late 1950s 'produced reductions in cervical cancer mortality of 60–70%
within 15 years'.[38]

The physical problems following treatment for cervical cancer in the
1960s and 1970s cannot be overlooked either. Radical hysterectomy and
radiotherapy both had serious side effects, physical and mental. Individuals
treated for cancer always live under a cloud: Will it return? Will I die? What
will happen to my family? Survivors were inevitably left with shortened,
scarred vaginas, often making sexual intercourse painful or impossible.
Radiation led to changes to the adjacent bowel and bladder, and sometimes
fistulous tracks between bowel, bladder and vagina, and incontinence. I
suspect most women would have preferred the 'mutilation' of hysterectomy
or vulvectomy to the enduring pain, suffering and death from cancer.

* * *

In her book Sandra Coney relates an episode that occurred early in 1988 and no doubt reflects the views of the postgraduate school and many members of the non-academic senior medical staff. She phoned an unnamed professor who had not attended the inquiry to ask if she could go to a lecture. He told her she would not be welcome: 'I'm controlling my anger towards you ... I've watched you destroy my colleague ... the staff here would be very resistant [to the removal of Professor Bonham]. You don't see the caring side of him.' He added that 'Green addressed a question [which] needed addressing'; the only thing he had done wrong was to 'go on for too long'. He was angry that 'a man of [Green's] age should have been subjected to an inquiry that did not provide "proper justice".[39]

When Coney contended that the hospital should have dealt with the issue 15 years before, the professor said he had 'been privy to all the debate and discussion over the years ... we decided to handle it in a gentlemanly way. We had great opportunities to attack McIndoe and McLean, but our ground rules were that it would not happen.' The 1984 paper was 'dishonest' and 'not a sound paper scientifically', and it 'was written to favour the view of the authors'. The media were also to blame. The whole thing was 'a battle in your [Coney's] overall strategy to destroy the hospital'.[40]

This was a remarkable exchange. Despite Bonham's protestations to the contrary at the inquiry, the unnamed professor admitted there had been longstanding discussions about Green's study within the academic department. I do not believe they had a gentlemen's agreement not to 'attack' McIndoe and McLean. They made no attempt to communicate with the journal editor about our 'dishonest' paper. They were scared stiff by the truth of its revelations and did not have the moral fibre to address them. The unnamed professor also raised with Coney the question of an 'inquiry into the inquiry'. I was aware that some of my colleagues had discussions with lawyers about the possible challenge to the findings of the inquiry; clearly this did not go ahead.

At one stage Valerie Smith, a family friend and neighbour of Green's for 25 years, attempted to instigate a judicial review of the inquiry and report, and in particular the judge's 'misrepresentation' of our 1984 paper. However, she eventually conceded that the grounds on which she relied had no substance, and she acknowledged via her counsel that she herself had misunderstood the judge's findings. She ultimately consented to the application by the attorney-general to strike out the proceedings. The Public Issues Committee of the Auckland District Law Society carefully examined the findings of the inquiry and concluded 'there is no evidence to suggest the Judge misinterpreted the McIndoe paper'.[41]

I was stung by the continuing public criticisms both of our papers and of me personally. I was also upset by the lack of support or contrition among my colleagues. Three years after publication of the Cartwright Report it became imperative, as a matter of public record, that I respond to their criticisms in the *New Zealand Medical Journal*. I first pointed out that there had been no criticisms of the 1984 paper until the inquiry in 1987. Even at the inquiry Bonham had said he had no evidence to show the methodology and conclusions of the 1984 paper could be challenged. But those who saw the inquiry as a threat to the hospital and senior colleagues needed to discredit the 1984 paper.

Regarding the criticism we had received for not publishing the paper in New Zealand, I pointed out that the material had been presented at the New Zealand Society of Pathologists' meeting in 1976 and the NWH Silver Jubilee Meeting two years later, and at international conferences in 1978, 1982 and 1984. On each occasion abstracts had been published. 'The prestigious nature of *Obstetrics and Gynecology* and its wide international circulation made it the ideal vehicle for dissemination of this unique material.' I stressed once again that we had given prepublication copies to the medical superintendent, the head of the postgraduate school, the head of the relevant clinical team and many other members of the senior medical staff.[42]

I had expected a brisk correspondence to result, but there were no responses in the *New Zealand Medical Journal*. Although I did receive a number of messages of personal support from senior members of the profession, none was prepared to commit their words to the public domain.

Some time after the inquiry I received an unexpected phone call from Wellington gynaecologist friend and former RNZCOG president Graeme Duncan. I had previously been a member of the college council and Duncan had earlier approached me to consider putting my name foward for an executive role. He asked, 'How are things going?' I do not recall my response, but I do recall what he went on to say. 'A friendly bit of advice, Ron. Things may change in the future, but I suggest you don't consider an executive position in the New Zealand College in the foreseeable future.'

This was fortuitous advice. My interests turned to the international scene and I became actively involved in the International Society for the Study of Vulvovaginal Disease and the International Federation for Cervical Pathology and Colposcopy, both organisations intimately involved in the study of the natural history and management of precancerous lesions in the lower genital tract. In due course I became president of the ISSVD and chairman of the Scientific Committee of the IFCPC.

CHAPTER 11

RIGHT OR WRONG: HEAL OR HARM

In those days we trusted people, colleagues, to behave ethically ...

BERNIE KYLE, 1990

OUR HEROES ARE USUALLY perceived to have no frailties, no flaws or faults. My schoolboy hero was the large-framed, brusque, bearded doctor who was said to be the best-known Victorian after Gladstone. Dr W.G. Grace cared for working-class folk in the west of England during the winter months, while in summer he overturned every known cricketing record. Only in recent years have I learned that this famed doctor had no qualms about intimidating umpires – there is even anecdotal evidence he may have been a match-fixer.[1]

Few professions are immune to embarrassment and public questioning over the upholding of professional standards and ethical conduct. Perhaps the earliest proven case of scientific fraud, and certainly the first to have a formal retraction, was reported in the *British Medical Journal* in 1916. An American physician working in the British Army described a 'delineator' that was claimed to be better than X-rays for depicting gunshot injuries. Investigations revealed that his claims were fraudulent.[2] The physician was tried by court martial and sentenced to death by firing squad, but later committed to penal servitude, dying a year later in prison. The details remain embargoed until 2017, but the story brings a macabre twist to the 1966 *New Yorker* magazine cartoon with the caption 'It's publish or perish, and he hasn't published.'

In late 1994, as a Fellow, I received two letters from the Royal College of Obstetricians and Gynaecologists of London. The first came from the president, Professor Geoffrey Chamberlain. 'There has,' he wrote, 'been a problem about two areas of research allegedly performed at St George's Hospital [of which he was head]. The results of these [two] quite separate research matters have been published in the *British Journal of Obstetrics and Gynaecology.*' He did not mention that he was editor-in-chief of the journal. He went on to say that, as a result of an inquiry, a consultant staff member – who, he also failed to mention, was a deputy editor of the same journal – had been suspended.

Chamberlain said newspapers had 'hinted at serious allegations some of which could be interpreted as involving [me] as Professor at St. George's Hospital', and ended by writing, '[S]peculation has been rife in the newspapers and much has not been based on fact.'[3] 'My name was put on the paper, and I agreed to it,' Chamberlain told the *British Medical Journal.* 'I have written to members of the college telling them that is the extent of my complicity. I had no part in the clinical part or the writing up of the paper. I was not involved in any deception.'[4] Professor Peter Rubin, head of the department of medicine at the University of Nottingham, told the *BMJ*: 'The practice of heads of department putting their names on papers with which they have had no involvement other than to create the environment in which the research took place is still more widespread than might be imagined.'[5]

Nine days later I received the second letter, explaining that Chamberlain had resigned as president of the college and editor-in-chief of the *British Journal of Obstetrics and Gynaecology.* An inquiry had found no evidence to support the findings of either of the research papers in question. Indeed, the case report to which the president's name was appended as co-author was entirely fictitious. The chairman of the investigating committee said Chamberlain had shown 'an error of judgment.'[6] Chamberlain had reached the pinnacle of his profession: president of a royal college, editor-in-chief of an international medical journal and a professor and head of his department – a potential candidate for a knighthood. To be charitable, perhaps his only misdemeanour was that he was too busy and too assured, both as professor and editor-in-chief, to consider there may have been major oversights in his performance in both roles. His real failing, though, was his attempt to dissociate himself from the events rather than saying honestly, 'I was stupid not knowing what was going on in my department and even more stupid to append my name to a scientific paper I knew nothing about', and apologising.

The policy of putting a head of department's name on a paper 'out of politeness' also extended to the antipodes. Michael Churchouse, as senior researcher and author of a particular paper in 1967, included the name of a research member of Bonham's department, Gary Carter, as an author.[7] Bonham's name was not included because he had played no active role in the study. But Bonham told Carter he wanted to be the lead author because he was head of department. Churchouse objected. Shortly afterwards Liggins visited Churchouse in his office and said, 'It would be politic to put Bonham's name on the paper, because if you don't, Carter will not have his contract renewed.' Churchouse recalled, 'This personally appalled me and to my innocent mind it seemed an immoral practice. I couldn't be the vehicle of Gary losing his job, so I said Bonham could be the third author.'[8]

The media, which delights in the activities of cheating sportsmen, deviant clerics, thieving lawyers and incompetent surgeons, also relishes the exposure of crooked scientists and unethical medical researchers. In a 1993 book entitled *Fraud and Misconduct in Medical Research*, New Zealand was marked as a country with 'active research programmes' that had 'not come to grips with the problem, though almost certainly it is present'.[9]

Nearly all agencies that have attempted to define scientific misconduct have used variations of the description adopted by the National Academy of Sciences: 'fabrication, falsification or plagiarism in proposing, performing or reporting research'.[10] There is a never-ending spectrum of reprehensible practices in science and in the behaviour of some scientists, and no definition will encompass all of these. How should we regard those individuals who deliberately turn a blind eye to medical or scientific misdemeanour? As one commentator has noted, 'Like a priest betraying a confession or a journalist revealing his source, a scientist who commits fraud violates a central principle of the perpetrator's profession.'[11]

It is a criminal offence to lie to the United States government, but a misstatement is a lie only if the person who made it can be shown to have *intended* to deceive. Rebecca Dresser, in an expert legal opinion, has addressed the confusion over the intent of the accused in scientific misconduct. She noted that those who analyse scientific misconduct frequently allude to 'culpable mental state' concepts, adopting phrases such as 'intent to deceive', 'unethical conduct' or 'knowing misrepresentation'. Some consider that the term 'scientific fraud' should replace 'scientific misconduct', on the grounds that 'fraud' more clearly conveys intent.[12]

Green's reclassification of the cases in his study unquestionably constituted scientific misconduct, though it is unlikely he considered it such. Harm was certainly done to some of his patients. The in-house working party should have identified the harm and stopped the experiment. So the question is, did Green *intend* to deceive?

As our understanding of ethics progresses, so too does the breadth of its terminology and semantics. Modern ethics has embraced a much broader intellectual framework, extending beyond ensuring patient safety to include concepts such as integrity, respectfulness, dignity, trust, transparency and justice. But letting go of strongly held beliefs is not easy. In *Researching with Integrity*[13] Bruce Macfarlane highlights a New Zealand example of the difficulties encountered by one researcher. On the basis of new research, in 1997 John Colquhoun abandoned 'a strongly held belief which formed part of [his] identity'. 'I now realise,' he wrote later, that

> what my colleagues and I were doing was what the history of science shows all professionals do when their pet theory is confronted by disconcerting new evidence: they bend over backwards to explain away the new evidence. They try very hard to keep their theory intact – especially so if their own professional reputations depend on maintaining that theory, and enthusiasts for a theory can fool themselves very often and persuade themselves and others that their activities are genuinely scientific.[14]

Also at work, perhaps, with Green's misguided stubbornness, is the theory of cognitive dissonance – the discomfort people feel when confronted with information that is inconsistent with their beliefs. Some, instead of acknowledging their error of judgement, reformulate their views in a new way in order to justify their old opinions.[15]

Although discussion of moral principles has existed since the beginning of civilisation, the ethical principles of human experimentation were subjected to closer scrutiny internationally only after the Nazi atrocities of World War II, and have become a respected discipline in more recent years. The principles of the Nuremburg Code (1947) were considered sufficiently important by the judges in the Doctors' Trial (the first of the 12 Nuremburg trials) to be used as a template against which some defendants were judged; an important provision concerned the requirements for consent.[16]

Green received approval for his ill-conceived and unethical experiment at a time when radical reforms in the field of human ethics were being instituted elsewhere, particularly in the United States. I do not recall any serious discussion on medical ethics or human experimentation when I was a student at the Otago Medical School in the mid-1960s, though medical etiquette was touched upon. On our first day we were reminded to demonstrate respect for the bodies in the dissection room, but human skeletons, including skulls, were traded as commodities, along with books, in the medical school exchange.

Striking parallels exist between the natural history studies of Green in Auckland and the widely reported Tuskegee study, which began in 1932 in Alabama and was conducted by the US Public Health Service. Over a period of 40 years, treatment was withheld from a group of 400 African-American men with syphilis. The aim was to compare the outcome of untreated syphilis in this group with an early twentieth-century Norwegian study among white European males. Both Green's and the Tuskegee study were driven by powerful men supported by senior colleagues – in the American case by no less a person than the surgeon-general. Dr Taliaferro Clark, the first Tuskegee investigator, described his study as an 'unparalleled opportunity for the study of the effect of untreated syphilis', while another opined that 'syphilis is not too bad a disease'.[17] Green said, 'If the physician does not worry too much about the disease then neither will the patient', and described his study as 'unique in the world'.[18]

Both studies ignored pre-existing evidence, were poorly planned and monitored, lacked formal protocols and were modified over time with the introduction of partial treatment. Participants were poorly educated African-American men, or mainly working-class women attending a public clinic. Most were unaware they were part of research programmes (the Tuskegee men were in fact lied to), were not given the opportunity to consent and had placed their trust in their attending doctors. Doctors not directly involved with the research were compliant with it or failed to institute changes in policy. Results from both studies were published regularly in medical journals.

Regarding the Tuskegee study, John Fletcher has pointed out the risks in judging the actions of earlier generations and concluded by asking whether reasonable, well-informed individuals would have excused Clark from the 'ordinary moral duty of honesty'. Doctors, he wrote, performed 'on' rather than 'with' uninformed participants. He also noted that there was never any intent to seek informed consent, but there was intent to disguise the experiments with medical beneficence, free care, partial treatment and false reassurance.[19] Despite years of attempts by McIndoe and McLean in New Zealand, and by Peter Buxton in the United States, to bring the respective experiments to an end, both were stopped only when they were exposed in the mainstream media.

There are parallels also between Green's behaviour and that of an early twentieth-century Austrian experimental biologist, Dr Paul Kammerer. Kammerer refused to accept the Darwinian view of evolution based on random selection. He believed instead that the main evolutionary vehicle was the 'inheritance of acquired characteristics' postulated by Jean-Baptiste Lamarck in 1809, and that useful adaptive changes in parents are preserved by heredity and transmitted to their offspring. Kammerer's experiments on the midwife toad (*Alytes obstetricians*) provided support for the Lamarckian argument, and drew upon him the 'full fury of the orthodox neo-Darwinians'. This movement was led by Professor William Bateson, the Cambridge Darwinian evolutionist who coined the word 'genetic'.

Kammerer's undoing was the nuptial pads – small coloured callosities – on the male midwife toad that gave him a better grip on the female during mating. Kammerer claimed these dark-coloured pads were proof of acquired characteristics; his opponents denied their existence. Finally it was revealed that the discolouration of the nuptial pads was not due to natural causes but to the injection of Indian ink. Following this disclosure Kammerer shot himself. His suicide was accepted as a confession of guilt, and his work was discredited. In his book *The Case of the Midwife Toad*, Arthur Koestler described Kammerer as 'sincere', 'a much-abused and lovable character' and 'honest although his results were phoney'[20] – comments that could equally be applied to Herbert Green.

A similar modern study of scientific fraud dates from 1974, when Dr William Summerlin, an immunologist in the prestigious Sloan Kettering Institute in New York, used a black pen to darken a transplanted black skin patch on two white mice. The scientific community regarded his behaviour as an aberration – so much so that he was sent on prolonged sick leave on full pay. An investigating committee later found he had lied and fabricated evidence, but when dismissing him they 'praised his personal qualities of warmth and enthusiasm'[21]

A striking feature of many reports of inquiry into scientific misconduct is the frequently apologist stance of the investigating committees, which often include colleagues. Rather than strongly condemning the research, they often praise unrelated qualities in the researcher.

Most New Zealand doctors in the mid-1960s were members of the New

Zealand branch of the London-based British Medical Association (BMA). In the 1965–66 British Medical Association *Annual Handbook*, 14 of the 15 pages devoted to medical ethics were allocated to the administration of the profession, including matters of etiquette such as the obligation of doctors one to another, complaints, discipline, advertising and publicity. The single page devoted to 'Ethical Obligations to Patients' deals largely with the doctors' ability to accept or refuse an individual as a patient, and the issue of professional discretion. The brief section on 'consent to examination or treatment' states: 'It is generally accepted that the appearance of a person for examination is indication of consent. It is however necessary to have a clear prior consent before embarking on treatment.' It goes on to say: 'What to tell a patient about his illness calls for discretion on the part of the doctor. There is no question the patient has a right to know the facts and the opinion of his case … [W]hen an opinion is demanded by the patient the doctor may deem it wise to discuss the situation with the relatives of how far he should go in this direction.'[22]

This makes it clear that in 1966 patients had the 'right to know the facts' – in this case that the standard management of CIS according to the hospital protocol was by cone biopsy – and that Green's intention was *not* to treat them. Had they asked for his 'opinion of the case' he is unlikely to have provided them with an honest, independent opinion, however, but his own 'atypical' viewpoint. Green's actions were clearly unethical. 'Doctor knows best' was the mantra; there was often no dialogue with patients on their involvement in teaching or research. The final sentence in the BMA handbook reads: 'Above all, [the BMA] relies on the character and conscience of its members.' As we have seen, Green repeatedly referred to his clear conscience.

US research institutions were just beginning to grapple with the issues. In 1965, when Green was planning his experiment, most members of the United States National Institutes of Health *ad hoc* committee reviewing research procedures endorsed a hands-off policy that gave investigators sole discretion in determining the risks and benefits to patients involved in experiments.[23] A seminal paper on 'Ethics and clinical research', by Henry Beecher of Harvard Medical School, was published in the *New England Journal of Medicine* in June 1966. Beecher summarised 22 'ethically objectionable' experiments, including four at the Harvard Medical School and three at the National Institutes of Health, where test subjects had been unable to give free consent. Beecher contended that 'Thoughtlessness and carelessness, not a wilful disregard of the patient's rights, accounts for the cases encountered ...'[24] Today we would regard Beecher's comments as a generous assessment; no doubt they reflected the prevailing opinion of the time. Beecher noted that 'the Nuremburg Code presents a rigid act of legalistic demand', while the 1964 'Declaration of Helsinki presents ethical guidelines and is therefore more broadly useful' and more closely reflects the realities of medical research. In regard to 'Non-Therapeutic Clinical Reseach' the Declaration of Helsinki states: '[C]linical research on a human subject cannot be undertaken without his [her] free consent after he [she] has been fully informed ...'[25]

Also in 1966 the US surgeon-general, together with the Public Health Service, issued a policy statement announcing that, for any research study, a review should be undertaken by 'a committee of institutional associates not directly associated with the project'.[26] This was made mandatory for all federally funded experimentation on humans, and for formal research grants. That same year, the Food and Drug Administration (FDA) ruled that, in the absence of informed consent, all experiments unrelated to therapy on human beings were forbidden.

While most advances in ethical thought were taking place in the United States, a controversial British physician, Maurice Pappworth, published *Human Guinea Pigs: Experimentation on man*, which described experiments in National Health Service hospitals and attracted vitriolic reviews; many academic colleagues were outraged by the book. The author was exiled from establishment London hospitals and waited 57 years to be elevated to fellowship of the Royal College of Physicians.[27]

One could be generous and say that Green was ignorant of the progressive moves taking place regarding clinical research in the United States. However, he was a young, widely read academic who travelled extensively and who was likely to have encountered such new opinion. He was familiar with the concepts of ethical practice and patient consent; he lectured and wrote about them in a 1958 paper on tubal ligation in the *New Zealand Medical Journal*:

> *Sterilisation for social or contraceptive reasons [is to be] viewed with great suspicion. Such cases constitute a subtle threat to the public welfare [and] are therefore illegal and unethical ... The doctor considering permanent sterilisation of a woman should always obtain at least one*

and preferably, two other opinions [and] have the full facts in writing
[and ensure] consent is fully and freely given without influence of
others.[28]

Interestingly, in the same year a fellow consultant at NWH laid a
formal complaint against Green for intervening in the care of one of his
patients who was about to undergo sterilisation. Green requested that the
anaesthetist stop the operation on the partially anaesthetised patient. The
patient, a 25-year-old woman, had severe congenital heart disease, one
living child, but only a single consultant's signature on the consent form.[29]

The issue relating to patient consent was established in a New Zealand
Court of Appeal judgement against one of Green's surgical colleagues in
1965. The Chief Justice, Sir Harold Barrowclough, ruled that 'if a doctor is
questioned about the possible consequences of a proposed treatment his
legal duty is to reply with "care and honesty".'[30] In a commentary on the
judgement, Peter Sim emphasised that the decision related only to situations
in which a patient questioned a doctor directly. It is unlikely any of Green's
patients would have challenged him with questions relating to risk. As Sim
also noted, 'there may be situations … where … the consensus of medical
opinion is that it is proper to warn a patient of risks, even without a specific
request for information.'[31] But in the 1960s few patients questioned their
treatment; they trusted and accepted the recommendations of their doctor.

Many New Zealand hospitals introduced *ad hoc* ethics committees
before these were formally mandated by the Health Department in 1972. The
NWH Medical Committee was 'responsible for the clinical organisation of
National Women's Hospital in order that … the professional and scientific
work shall be properly carried out therein.'[32] The phrase 'properly carried
out' implies an ethical duty of which patient safety is a central component.

Much later Tony Baird, as chairman of the NZMA Central Ethics
Committee, claimed:

> *It is not true that the women who took part in the study by Associate*
> *Professor Green knew nothing about it. The Inquiry heard only from*
> *the women who were complaining about the study. The women saw*
> *medical staff other than Green and, as a registrar and tutor specialist,*
> *I saw women who not only knew about their participation in the study*
> *but were happy with what was happening to them. Some of these women*
> *volunteered that they would like to have been heard at the Inquiry but*
> *were deemed not to be suitable for it.*[33]

Judge Cartwright's contemporaneous notes tell a different story:

> *I wrote to all Group 2 women encouraging them to meet me to discuss matters relevant to the inquiry and a number of these women indicated their willingness to do this. I also publicly asked for any women patients with abnormal smears who had been treated at National Women's to contact me. Extensive publicity was given to this request, particularly through local radio stations and newspapers, and as a consequence a large number of women contacted me by telephone or wrote to me.*[34]

Of the 44 women who were interviewed by Cartwright, 'only one woman knew that she had been included in a research project. Many, including "Ruth", believed they had been used as guinea pigs, but equally some, when they spoke to me, were of the view that they had been offered generally accepted treatment.' Cartwright further observed: 'After reading the files and listening to their experiences I could only conclude that the vast majority of people I talked to had so little knowledge of the condition for which they or their relatives were being monitored that they had no basis from which to formulate a complaint.'[35]

How much risk are women with a gynaecological cancer prepared to accept? A recent Australian study compared women's attitudes to the possibility of cancer cells being 'missed'. They were offered a less radical operation for early-stage vulval cancer, or a more radical procedure from which there was a 60 per cent chance they would develop permanently swollen legs. Despite this risk, 80 per cent of women chose the more radical operation if there was a greater than one in 100 risk that cancer cells would be 'missed' by the lesser procedure.[36] Clearly, women are not prepared to accept even very small risks in the management of their cancer. Yet Green almost certainly did not discuss the risks of his experiment with the women involved.

Some of Judge Silvia Cartwright's harshest comments were directed at the failure of the medical profession. Despite 'increasing opposition to the 1966 trial, both internationally and at National Women's Hospital, there was no will to confront the difficult issues [that] emerged. For twenty years there was criticism, yet no special effort was made to ensure that patients' health did not suffer as a result of Dr Green's attempt to prove his hypothesis … The medical profession failed in its basic duty to its patients.'

Cartwright suggested that doctors confused 'ethics with etiquette'.[37] This story is not solely of Green's blind adherence to a flawed, unethical experiment; it is also the story of misplaced professional loyalty in a rigidly hierarchical system that prevented the application of sound ethical principles. Eliot Friedson has argued that medicine's claims to 'ethicality' are little more than rhetoric designed to justify privilege and power, unless the profession can genuinely deliver the service it professes in its code of ethics.[38]

* * *

I am sometimes asked, 'Could the unfortunate experiment happen today?' I hope not, but, given the frailty of the human condition, my answer is a qualified yes. Following final approval, research projects are rarely monitored independently. During its course an experiment can change in both emphasis and direction. As we have seen in Green's experiment, individuals can impose their personalities and names, and the commercialisation of educational institutes such as universities has increased the pressure to publish. Majorities may, on occasion, be swayed by powerful minorities. On the other hand, consensus is not a guide to scientific truth. There are endless opportunities for scientific fraud.

When Professor Neville Hacker was asked if Australian women could suffer such an unfortunate experiment, he replied,

The New Zealand experience is a salutary lesson for us all. It demonstrates the problems the profession has with self-regulation, and with the accountability of individual members. In spite of Quality Assurance, ethics committees and all other attempts at internal regulation, doctors in positions of power and influence can be very difficult for the profession to control, [particularly] if the ideas they propagate are misguided, albeit well-intentioned.[39]

(It is sobering to reflect that if modern ethics committees had existed when McLean, McIndoe and I were preparing our 1984 paper we might not have been able to carry out our research for the article, because the patients were not our own and we did not have ethics committee approval.[40])

Whose responsibility was it to intervene and stop Green's experiment? Quite clearly it was initially Bonham's. He had been aware of the outcome of Green's experiment for some years but had chosen to do nothing about it. Next, responsibility fell to the other senior members of the academic department: as Cartwright pointed out, they chose to 'avoid the issue', even following publication of our paper. After them, responsibility lay with the non-academic doctors at NWH, especially those working with Green. In the end, it was left to those of us at the bottom of the hospital hierarchy to blow the whistle.

Jeremy Hopkins, one-time chairman of the New Zealand Medical Association and its Ethics Committee, described 1988 as 'surely … the watershed year in the history of New Zealand medicine'.[41] He might have added that, while medical ethics as a discipline lagged behind clinical medicine, the moral compass of right or wrong, and 'do no harm', should have guided clinicians along the correct path.

Professor Barbara Heslop and Dr Alan Gray, representing the Cancer Society of New Zealand, also pointed out in 1989:

There was no system (and still isn't) that would allow Drs McIndoe, McLean and Warren to have Professor Green's research independently reviewed at least 15 years before the Inquiry, when they asked for it, and when a review might have prevented unnecessary deaths. Not a very proud record for either the University, the Auckland Hospital Board, or the Department of Health, who must take final responsibility for what happened at National Women's Hospital.[42]

Dr Jim Rossiter, who blew the whistle on academic fraudster Michael Briggs, has eloquently described my own views:

I am struck by the inability of many individuals to accept that a senior person is dishonest; by the attacks on personal integrity in a situation where the recipient is unable to reply; and by the behaviour of people commanding respect in the community who say one thing in private and another in public. The price of exposing fraud and deceit is high; it is sad, but necessary, that all stages of research must be guarded by vigilant people who must act without fear of the consequences of what they do.[43]

The 'unfortunate experiment' at NWH rates, with Tuskegee, as one of the worst examples of known human experimentation, outside of war, in the twentieth century.

CHAPTER 12

MABEL'S STORY

[Green's] disciples have a uniquely blind faith.

Dr Dan O'Connor

The influence of Green's expertise and professional position on both women and doctors was far reaching. Women were referred to him from other parts of New Zealand and some even travelled from overseas to consult with him.

Immediately following a consultation with a patient, Green would dictate his impressions of the visit in the patient's notes. These records of his spontaneous thoughts often reveal considerable insight into his sometimes irrational thinking and his lack of regard for the long-term welfare of the women under his care.

An Australian colleague of mine forwarded copies of the records of one of Green's patients, Mabel (not her real name), the wife of a doctor, and discussed with me the management of her condition. She was the second patient he had seen who had been 'grossly mismanaged by Green'. Mabel's records provide a further chilling commentary on how Green's erroneous views affected not only the patient and her family but also doctors beyond New Zealand. As my colleague noted, 'one of the things which amazed me to the end was the way in which her husband was totally persuaded by Herb Green to accept his philosophy. This from a doctor.'[1]

In 1969 a general surgeon in New Zealand performed a cervical smear on Mabel at the same time as he assessed her for haemorrhoid surgery. The smear was abnormal and the surgeon performed a cone biopsy on the cervix at the time of her haemorrhoidectomy. The pathology report recorded: 'The *in-situ* lesion extends for the full depth of the lesion.' A follow-up smear was abnormal and her gynaecologist referred her to Green for a second opinion regarding further management. A colposcopy examination in Auckland with McIndoe revealed a 3–4cm lesion consistent with CIS in a segment extending from the cervix onto the upper vagina.

Green observed:

We do not think in this hospital that it [CIS] is significant as regards the possible development of invasive carcinoma and ... it can be safely left without further operative or irradiation treatment ... we think these lesions ultimately regress and ... there is no danger of an invasive cancer developing ... there is no necessity for a check-up more than yearly and to make examinations more often than this induces unwarranted mental trauma in the mind of the patient.

CIS can extend from the cervix onto the adjacent vagina and treatment involves excision of all abnormal skin. Vaginal CIS is relatively uncommon and although its natural history was not clearly established in the 1960s, the general principle existed that *in-situ* lesions were premalignant and should be eradicated. There was no evidence that such lesions regressed. Green had begun another natural history study. Given the relative rarity of vaginal CIS, it is unlikely Green had experience in the 'conservative' management of the condition. His decision not to treat Mabel had no rational basis.

A year later, asked to advise on Mabel's continuing smear abnormalities, Green noted that McIndoe's cytology confidently reported the cells to be 'sinister'. For a man with generally assured opinions on this subject, his response, to Mabel's gynaecologist, was now less than confident: 'I am not very sure how to advise you but only to say we have our problems in this direction also ... we would have a look with the colposcope, and try to pick out a suitable area for biopsy.' The only reason for a further biopsy would have been to exclude an early cancer.

When Mabel visited Green again in October 1972 he noted, 'We have had pathology problems recently ... she was asymptomatic and there was ... no clinical evidence of anything [which] could be construed as suspicious.' He was unable to examine the cervix adequately because of scarring from her previous cone biopsy. With the aid of the colposcope Green observed an extension of the lesion on the vagina to 4–5cm, and a biopsy again confirmed CIS. However, he was opposed to 'the mutilating and potentially dangerous operation of total colpectomy [vaginectomy], and deep X-ray treatment' and proposed to 'do nothing. The process has gone on now for so long ... this is the sensible thing to do. On the basis of my personal experience with this type of lesion I cannot imagine anything serious happening within 15 years ... I have put these alternatives as plainly as I could to the Dr and [Mabel] and I think they have accepted the third alternative.'

Early in 1974 Mabel's Wellington gynaecologist reported to Green that he had had to perform a hysterectomy because of a pyometra – her uterus was enlarged with pus, a consequence of obstruction of the cervix by scar tissue from the previous operations on her cervix. Green observed that she would continue to have abnormal smears.

In 1975 the gynaecologist decided to refer Mabel to a radiotherapist, noting that she had seen Green in Auckland:

As you know he is conducting a conservative clinic in which they hang on to these people on the assumption ... the life cycle does not go on to cancer. Well she went on and on and very little change took place except that it [the smear] was always Grade 4 ... the 64-dollar question is what to do with this. Do we just sit back and wait? ... We have been sitting on her since 1969.

The radiotherapist recommended the application of an anticancer cream, 5-fluorouracil, in the vagina.

A year later Mabel again consulted Green following a further biopsy finding of probable invasive vaginal cancer. Green wrote, 'Both Jock McLean and I have looked at the slides and both consider it cannot be called invasive cancer.' In an independent response to the pathologist, however, McLean gave a rather different interpretation.

We [Green and McLean] have been incommunicado over the last few years because of my criticisms of his excursions into pathology – without too much success. I call this [biopsy] probable carcinoma in-situ of the vaginal vault.

We have had, over the years, about a dozen or so patients with this sort of lesion. Herb has been trying to say that these vaginal vault lesions are harmless and do not progress to invasive carcinoma, as he has been saying with carcinoma in-situ of the cervix. In actual fact, some have progressed to invasive carcinoma and I think, from memory, two have died from invasive cancer ... These patients have generally been treated conservatively until it is too late.

I hope the clinician looking after [Mabel] has not been lulled into a false sense of security on the question of the potential sinisterness of this lesion.

Green remained unmoved: 'Only in the last resort, in the presence of unequivocal clinical evidence, should you resort to radiation.'

Mabel and her husband moved to Australia, where they consulted two experienced gynaecological cancer surgeons. According to Green, both specialists 'seemed to be alarmed' and one 'was quite surprised when I said I had several such cases and … the only ones [who] got into trouble had been the ones treated with radiation.' The surgeon had 'recommended surgical or radiation treatment … he … had not much experience in the conservative management of this type of lesion'.

Mabel and her husband returned to New Zealand, where Mabel had a further biopsy and again sought Green's opinion. He observed that while the New Zealand pathologist said 'there was unequivocal evidence of invasive cancer … I would strongly disagree with her'.

Green commented on his naked-eye inspection, noting grossly abnormal vaginal skin now extending the length of the vagina to the external urethra, and went on to say: 'I had a fairly long discussion with the Dr and his wife about how to manage the lesion and did my best to reassure them that what experience I have convinces me … it is not of serious import – unless it is treated by radiation … which they are both totally unwilling to consider.'

Green had no mandate to observe vaginal CIS without treatment. Once again, he recorded the progressive extension over 10 years of a small, treatable CIS lesion until it covered the entire vagina, making management progressively more difficult. He disagreed with the pathologist's diagnosis of cancer – and was ultimately proven wrong. He finally admitted in a letter to one of the Australian surgeons, 'It is clinically developing a malignant course.'

A year later Mabel returned to Green with bleeding. His notes recorded that the lesion was 'undoubtedly progressing as shown by its clinical features and I think the time has come to consider radiation treatment. I hesitated to do so in the past in similar cases because of the fear that true malignancy would be precipitated but recent review of such cases convinces me … malignancy is inevitable if it is not irradiated.'

Mabel eventually accepted Green's advice to have radiotherapy. As the radiotherapist noted, 'This treatment, which I regard as somewhat inadequate, has been dictated to me by both Professor Green and her husband, [as] I would normally place a small radium applicator in the vault.' Green's powers of persuasion clearly influenced Mabel's doctor/ husband, who supported Green to the end.

When *in-situ* lesions involve additional organs such as the cervix, the vagina and/or the vulval/perineal region, each lesion is managed on an individual basis, while taking cognisance of the whole. Mabel subsequently had further surgery to the vulva for premalignancy, but ultimately died of pelvic cancer, which had probably originated in the region of the cervix and upper vagina.

If Green's 'natural history studies' on Mabel and Phoebe – and many other similar cases – had not convinced him that CIS is a precancer, nothing would. Phoebe and Mabel and the others had been unwitting victims of an experiment based on a whim and a misbelief. Green's wilful blindness to the sometimes distressing symptoms; his misinterpretation or dismissal of the findings of the pathology examinations; his determination to cling to a misguided belief in the face of glaring evidence – all contributed to the suffering of his patients and their families.

CHAPTER 13

A PROFESSION DIVIDED

I have borne a burden of guilt for not having seen the study
for what it was at the outset.

Mont Liggins

THE MEDICAL SYSTEM OF the 1960s that nurtured me as a medical student and young doctor, in both New Zealand and Britain, was patriarchal, hierarchical and largely autonomous. Academic doctors determined the content of medical training; medico-political doctors defined the nature and quality of medical work and discipline; etiquette was more important than ethics; clinical freedom was more important than scientific evidence; senior surgeons and physicians 'knew best'; there was no multidisciplinary 'team' approach to patient care as there is today; and the profession ensured that paramedical practitioners played a subservient role.

Although the central ethos of medicine was to provide patient care, a subtext was that patients in public hospitals could be 'used' for teaching and research, often without their consent or even their knowledge. As late as 1979, Dr Frank Rutter, chairman of the Auckland Hospital Board, said women 'had a moral obligation to allow their bodies to be used for teaching purposes'.[1] The era of 'honoraries' (unpaid consultants) doling out benevolence at their whim was over, but such attitudes still persisted. A minority of consultants were arrogant, patronising and intimidating to students, young doctors and patients alike.

There were a number of overlapping hierarchies: academic, with titles; years of service; and specialty – senior physicians and senior surgeons ranked above other specialists. Progress up the training ladder relied on satisfactory personal references and, finally, professional examinations. At the bottom of the ladder were house surgeons and registrars; further up were junior and middle-grade specialists; above them, a small number of specialists who were designated 'seniors' by hospital boards. Selection for seniority depended on years of service, leadership qualities and medico-political standing. The conferral of seniority status was worthy of newspaper comment. Seniority carried not only a better salary but, more importantly, status in the profession. Those who had attained this status determined the career prospects of those below them, and happily for them, were excluded from the 'on call' roster. Maintaining a good relationship with 'seniors' was a priority if one were to progress up through the system. Failure to support – or speaking out against – policies promoted by more senior staff potentially compromised career prospects.

Most academic units had one 'full' professor who was also the head of the department – a position usually held until retirement. NWH was an exception: Bonham, Liley and Liggins were all professors, as was, later, Mantell. Green was an associate professor. In the 1960s there was no love lost between medical superintendent Dr Algar Warren and the senior academics, who tolerated but largely dominated him. Power was entrenched in the senior academic and a few senior non-academic clinicians, who made all the important decisions.

Twice a week the hospital observed the classic, time-honoured ritual. Miss Verna Murray, the matron, in her immaculate starched white uniform and stiff, tent-like veil, presented an imposing figure when escorting Algar Warren as they strode through the corridors to confer with staff, reassure patients and admire newborn babies.

From childhood I recognised that doctors enjoyed an elevated social position in the community; they were to be trusted and respected. Many, especially specialists, attained a godlike aura; some were distant and unapproachable. Family connections in medicine were important. A doctor's son in my medical school class told me, in complete sincerity, that since my father was a freezing worker, I might 'struggle'. In Christchurch in the 1960s almost all surgeons came from the 'right school' and were, more often than not, appointed to fill their fathers' shoes. During my time in England I was aware that most doctors came from upper-middle-class professional backgrounds. My colleague Dr Mike Hambly told me of his pre-entry interview with the Dean of St Bartholomew's Hospital Medical School in 1960, which coincided with a dockers' strike in the nearby Port of London. 'The Dean, aware I was from a line of medical men, enquired whether I thought I should receive preferential entry. I said I didn't think this was appropriate. The Dean responded, "If you can become a docker only if your father is a docker, why shouldn't it be the same for entry to this medical school?'"[2] Society was changing rapidly; women were beginning to enter the professions and feminism was advancing. A new social order in New Zealand was increasingly affording children from working-class backgrounds the opportunity to study medicine. But when I returned to New Zealand in 1973, my illusion of an egalitarian senior medical staff was dashed by the powerful tribal hierarchy I encountered at NWH.

I was grateful to be appointed directly to a junior specialist position and was soon absorbed without fuss into the lowest rank of the specialist hierarchy, supporting the status quo and demonstrating unswerving loyalty to the system that had placed me there. Over time I became increasingly conscious of the subtle power and intellectual intimidation exerted by some members of the senior academic staff, and this irked me. There were occasions when, against my better judgement, I allowed myself to be subjected to intimidation and even blackmail. I regret now that I did not stand up more forcefully to subtle bullying. My first three years were in a temporary position and I was anxious to obtain a permanent consultant post, so, like many members of the lower echelons, I found it was easiest to avoid hospital politics. This was at the time McIndoe and McLean were battling in the Senior Medical Staff Committee with their concerns over Green's experiment in the hospital – they could have done with my support.

Teaching and research were driving influences at NWH. Green set himself up as the national authority on CIS of the cervix and had ample opportunities to expound his views. The more he wrote and lectured, the more of an expert he became in his own eyes and also those of his colleagues and students. He did not rate McIndoe, the only man in the hospital with comparable knowledge of CIS. And his strong personality meant he had no qualms in exercising his power and position to intimidate those, including me, who challenged him. Some doctors cope poorly with conflict and with colleagues who hold strong alternative opinions. Naturally, Green's presentations to medical audiences were designed to make them follow his line of thinking. Many doctors were influenced by his rejection of the concept of routine cervical screening. As Dr Alan Gray has noted, 'Dr Green was a powerful influence in teaching in New Zealand – a small country often dominated by single-minded individuals on particular issues.'[3]

Bonham and Green were men from opposite ends of the earth, men from markedly different backgrounds, men with a curious mixture of qualities and defects, but in many ways men with similar natures. Both were ambitious, with strong opinions and difficult personalities. They were products of an era of patriarchal, professional males, many of whom sought positions of leadership and power. As C. Wright Mills has stated,

> *The power elite is composed of men whose positions enable them to transcend the ordinary environments of ordinary men and women; they are in positions to make decisions having major consequences. Whether they do or do not make such decisions is less important than the fact that they do occupy such pivotal positions: their failure to act, their failure to make decisions, is itself an act that is often of greater consequence than the decisions they do make.*[4]

Bonham's 'failure to act ... to make decisions' when he was well aware of the adverse outcomes from Green's experiment was the primary event that led to his downfall. Ultimately, the failure of these two men – the professor and the associate professor, the director and the deputy director, the victor and the vanquished – to establish a professional relationship led to a chain of failures that affected thousands of New Zealand women and extended over two generations. Both men basked in the international approbation their department was receiving from the ground-breaking research of their colleagues, Liley and Liggins. Sadly, Bonham and Green both ended up on the wrong side of history.

They were also bullies, like a lot of their male contemporaries – Prime Minister Robert Muldoon was a classic example. Bullying of an intellectually intimidatory kind was perceived to be necessary in order to shore up positions of power and influence – particularly in rigid, less transparent, bureaucratic hierarchies such as universities and hospitals. Sister Isobel Fisher remembered McIndoe avoiding Green in Ward 9; Ian Ronayne recalled intervening physically between Green and McIndoe, fearing the use of physical force by the former.

I never heard Green use the phrase 'clinical freedom', and it does not appear in his writings, but his actions clearly point to his belief in the divine right of doctors to do whatever they felt was best for their patients. Following the Cartwright Inquiry, a University of Auckland subcommittee addressing the Cartwright Report stressed that 'when people's health – and lives – [are] at stake academic independence must take second place to patient welfare.[5] As cardiologist J.R. Hampton had written in 1983, 'In days when investigation was non-existent and treatment as harmless as it was ineffective, the doctor's opinion was all there was. Clinical freedom was at least a cloak for ignorance and at worst an excuse for quackery – now clinical freedom is dead and no one need regret its passing.'[6]

In his book *In Sickness and in Power*, Dr David Owen, a co-founder of the British Social Democratic Party, explores the meaning of the Greek-derived word 'hubris' in relation to a number of powerful political leaders. He defines it as the supreme arrogance that leads some humans to think they are infallible.[7] Owen suggests the character traits that point to an individual with the 'hubris syndrome'. These include excessive confidence in one's own judgement; contempt for the advice of others; exaggerated self-belief; a conviction that, rather than being accountable to the court of one's colleagues, one answers to history or God; loss of contact with reality, often associated with progressive isolation from colleagues; a tendency to allow a 'broad vision', especially a conviction about the moral rectitude of a proposed course of action, to obviate the need to consider other aspects of it, such as an unwanted outcome; a wooden-headed refusal to change course; and a contempt for the opinion of others. Nearly all of these traits fitted Green. A combination of hubris, scientific fundamentalism and clinical freedom gave him free rein.

Leo Koss, who trained as a gynaecologist, became fascinated by the emerging field of cytology and was familiar with Green's views through his own studies of the natural history of cervical cancer. We became professional friends and one night, over dinner at his Manhattan apartment, discussed Green's experiment. He believed Green was well intentioned but took advantage of his position as the New Zealand authority on CIS and imposed his views on the local community.

There were other factors at work. NWH was isolated geographically. Both the old Cornwall and the new hospital were at some distance from the main Auckland Hospital and opportunities for interspecialty exchanges were limited. Although Greenlane General Hospital was close by, there was little interaction between the respective senior medical staffs. Had Green presented his proposal to the combined senior medical staffs of the Auckland hospitals in 1966 there is a strong probability it would have been rejected in its original form. After all, there were many astute physicians, surgeons and pathologists working in other specialties who dealt with *in-situ* cancers in other tissues. Some would have been familiar with the biological potential and risks of untreated *in-situ* lesions.

* * *

Loyalty to our family, friends and society is usually a virtue, but when it is misplaced, people suffer. And misplaced loyalty is central to the medical community's response to the 'unfortunate experiment'. At the outset none of Green's colleagues sincerely believed CIS was an innocent condition; no one in the world did. Yet from apathy and a sense of loyalty to their friend and colleague, they voted in favour of his flawed experiment. Bruce Grieve, the 'strongest' of the 'seniors', told a concerned McIndoe he felt 'prepared to allow Professor Green to proceed'.[8] Many years later at the inquiry Grieve said he was not 'absolutely positive' that CIS was a cancer precursor, yet he insisted on the inclusion of a clause in the proposal ensuring that his private patients 'were retained under my care for treatment'.[9]

In the words of John Fletcher, 'Moral sensitivity can be overwhelmed by excessive loyalty to the welfare of an institution [or an individual] and one's role within it. Strong and uncritical loyalty to an institution and role impair independence of observation, judgement and actions, especially to prevent or moderate conflicts of loyalty and conflicts of interest.'[10]

Kyle's suggestion of an independent investigation was vetoed in favour of an in-house working party. Alastair Macfarlane, the chairman, was a gentleman and an excellent clinician but lacked the necessary skills to deal with difficult professional conduct by a longstanding colleague. Bruce Faris, a friend and contemporary of Green's, was an opinionated old-school committee man. It became clear during the inquiry that he had not fully understood the 1966 proposal. He was unable to make an independent assessment of the study and to the end maintained blind loyalty to Green and the hospital. Professor Dick Seddon, originally a student of Green's, a resident medical officer under him and later a consultant with him on the academic team, was a fine doctor and a thoroughly good man. Soon after his appointment to the working party he accepted the chair of obstetrics and gynaecology in Wellington and from that time his mind was, no doubt, on his new role. Like Macfarlane, he was not comfortable about making the tough call. My view is that these three men were too close and too loyal to Green to be completely objective and independent, and I believe they failed to address the central concern: patient safety.

Over time, positions hardened and other staff were drawn in. Sustaining the reputation of the postgraduate school and maintenance of the established hierarchy within the hospital became paramount: patients were forgotten; moral principle was sacrificed for loyalty.

I have some sympathy for Green's colleagues who, in the 1960s and early 1970s, unwittingly became collateral damage of the 'unfortunate experiment' and the public inquiry. At the time doctors implicitly trusted the motives and actions of their colleagues; patients trusted their doctors. Hospitals functioned as extended families – not the businesses they are today; colleagues were, more often than not, close friends. Even today, professional friendships can blur objectivity and judgement.

I cannot, however, extend the same benevolence to my own colleagues. Why have some of my generation taken such strong 'defend and deny' positions regarding the matters that came before the Cartwright Inquiry? Why have some been such strong supporters of the revisionist viewpoint? Why have the majority remained silent? I can only assume they view loyalty to old colleagues and the profession as more important than their duty to patients, and that makes it impossible for them to apologise.

Dr Alan Gray has noted

Dr Green was a powerful influence in teaching in New Zealand – a small country often dominated by single-minded individuals on particular issues. ... It is a tragedy [the National Women's Hospital] has been brought to its knees by one man's total disregard for scientific method, the long term welfare of his patients, and his contempt for his colleagues. Many other doctors in this country to some extent share some part of the blame – they knew ... Dr Green was wrong and yet [they] were unwilling to do anything about it.[11]

The failure of the Cartwright Inquiry to acknowledge the unique contributions of NWH to the health of New Zealand women and children (although this, of course, was not its brief) served to fuel the antagonism of the medical profession towards its findings. So too did the widely published photograph of Silvia Cartwright with Coney, Bunkle and Clare Matheson ('Ruth') at a seminar a year later. Green's experiment and its consequences destroyed New Zealand's only national and international 'centre of excellence' in women's health. It was a pity that Judge Cartwright did not stress enough that the 'unfortunate experiment' was a significant medical failure brought about by a small group of very powerful academic medical men.

* * *

The very traditional male medical environment in which Green was so dominant was challenged by the feminism that was well established in New Zealand by the 1970s and 1980s. Older doctors were generally uneasy and uncertain about what feminism actually meant and how it would affect them and their women patients. Bonham held liberal and progressive views (for example, on the role of women doctors) but Green was a traditionalist. McIndoe, although excited that our paper was attracting attention, also expressed anxiety about Coney and Bunkle's approach. What were these women doing? What would they write? What would be the outcome? Doctors felt threatened by their challenges. But the feminists taught us many things, especially about the power of the pen and the media to disseminate sometimes unwelcome news.

1975, the year the NWH in-house subcommittee was set up, was also International Women's Year. This was a catalyst for the New Zealand Conference on Women and Health, organised jointly by the Committee on Women and the Department of Health, and held in 1977. The conference addressed 'enormous areas of serious concern and widespread evidence of underprivilege, exploitation and male domination of women worldwide … this conference is concerned to determine in what ways the medical system and the medical establishment contributed to, and reinforced, [women's] inferior position' in society.[12] Dr John Hiddlestone, director-general of health, agreed it was 'time to take stock and review the problem relating to women and health'. His views at that time were typical of the views of many individuals of both genders when he went on to say, 'I still believe … women's essential role is as wives, mothers and homemakers.'[13] Green would have applauded these sentiments. Phillida Bunkle observed that 'women remained as "outcasts" in the health services … power, policy-making and planning were, however, retained exclusively in the hands of a small group of male doctors and … the medical profession had assumed a form of moral authority in order to reinforce their position.'[14]

For Professor Barbara Heslop, the conference was mainly about power.

The women doctors [who attended], who might have been expected to be warmly accepted, found themselves not personae gratae *at all – they were accused of joining the men ... [and] the small group of women doctors at the meeting was, I think, rather shocked to hear of their shortcomings, although I take the point about the power of doctors, [and] the medical establishment fiddled away, blissfully unaware ... a lot of women had had enough of them and ... some were very angry. [It was difficult] to believe ... so many male and female antennae and so many hypothetical receptors could have remained in sleep mode for as long as they did. It was very late when some of them woke up.*[15]

Implementation of the 118 recommendations from the conference progressed slowly over the following decade, but everything was to change with the Cartwright Inquiry.

Coney, a knowledgeable journalist, and Bunkle, an academic feminist, were both experienced in bringing issues to the attention of the public. Unencumbered by professional loyalties, they were anxious to advance feminism and feminist health causes, determined to 'break the power' of a 'small group of male doctors' and committed to wresting from the medical profession 'the moral authority [that] reinforce[d] their position ... the things at stake were too important to let etiquette stand in the way'.[16]

I give Coney and Bunkle full credit for bringing the 'unfortunate experiment' to public attention. At no time did McIndoe, McLean or I consider approaching the media. We had brought the matter to the attention of our senior colleagues and the profession at large and we believed the leaders of the profession would rectify the problem. How wrong we were.

In one sense Coney and Bunkle were coming from the same direction as McIndoe, McLean and me – we all wanted a public depiction of the truth. In another sense, though, we were poles apart: they wanted an immediate and resounding victory; we were concerned about the future. Coney and Bunkle constituted a well-prepared unit with a committed following. They were single-minded, with prepared questions and tape recorder in hand. They appeared to have little interest in the future of NWH which, although battered and bruised, had to continue providing free medical services to the women of Auckland. Ironically, Coney's dramatic tactics drove women who could least afford it into private care. McLean was aware of the possible problems. As he told Coney, 'It's like dropping an atomic bomb on Hiroshima; you've done it and now we've got to build on it.'[17]

In an article aptly titled 'The speculum bites back', Auckland feminist Pat Rosier noted that the Cartwright Inquiry had 'international importance as an example of a feminist challenge to patriarchal medical structures', pointedly observing that our 1984 paper 'was written by three male doctors'.[18]

* * *

Could Green have been right? Was he being misjudged? Was the issue one of a personality clash with McIndoe and McLean? A case with a New Zealand connection illustrates this dilemma. Dr Wendy Savage, who held strongly voiced alternative views on women's health, upset some conservative colleagues when she worked as an obstetrician and gynaecologist in Gisborne in the mid-1970s. Following her return to the London Hospital, her academic chief, Professor Jurgis Grudzinskas, laid charges of incompetence against her. A leading article in the *British Medical Journal* noted: 'The most difficult problem in terms of competence occurs when one consultant has developed an individual approach to the management of his or her patients [which] is out of line with the views of others. If this view is sincerely held, thought through, and supported by published evidence, it cannot be described as incompetent but it will cause difficulties.'[19]

Savage stood up and fought, and was subsequently cleared. Although often controversial, she was not incompetent; the central issue was an irreconcilable clash of personalities. Such a clash was also present between Green and McIndoe, though McIndoe would have been right to perceive that Green was incompetent as well. McIndoe's premature death denied him the opportunity to vindicate his stance at the inquiry. Following Bonham's enforced retirement there were suggestions that Savage be appointed the new postgraduate professor at NWH.

There are further parallels with the Savage case. As the *British Medical Journal* observed, 'London University and the Royal College of Obstetricians and Gynaecologists, both of whom were well aware of the conflict well before it came to a head, might ask themselves whether their studied refusal to become involved might not have been mistaken. Someone somewhere should have acted sooner.'[20]

By the time of his last major report in 1974, Green had written 10 papers on the natural history of CIS. At the time he reported 'a series of 750 cases of *in-situ* cancer in which ten or 1.3% progressed to invasion, but there were only two in which there was no clinical or histological doubt about progression'. In other words he did admit that two cases progressed to cancer, but in the other eight cases the problem (according to Green) was either 'failure to exclude invasion at the outset or the over-diagnosis at a later stage'. He went on to say that his earlier views were 'perhaps overstated and must be modified, not because of a "rash" of invasive cancers but mainly because of the inability to exclude adequately diagnosed invasive cancer at the outset'.[21]

Green's argument was wrong. As described earlier, he removed cases before publication that he believed were 'missed' invasive cancers. The eventual diagnoses of cancer in his published series had nothing to do with 'missed' pathology diagnoses. If this were true, cancers would have started to appear sooner. His 1966 proposal depended on being able to exclude invasive cancer at the beginning; now he was saying that he could not do this. Surely this was the time for him to reappraise and to stop his experiment? Yet he persisted by writing: 'it does not seem [carcinoma in-situ] is a very dangerous lesion'.[22]

Although a minority – mainly epidemiologists – initially shared Green's views about screening, these opinions were untenable by the mid- to late 1960s. Leo Koss considered that Green 'held on to his views too long'.[23] Another professional colleague, Canadian epidemiologist Professor Anthony Miller, made a similar observation – 'the problem with Green was that he continued to observe when prudence dictated action'.[24] As Knox had noted, 'the cost in delays in instituting treatment resulted in lost lives'.[25]

Did Green ultimately consider he might have been wrong? Having written approximately one paper a year between 1962 and 1974 on the natural history of CIS, he suddenly stopped reporting his findings. Was he having second thoughts? The cessation of his publishing could not have been, as he suggested, because he knew McIndoe was intending to publish: McIndoe's initial abstract was not published until 1979, and our definitive paper came five years later. Although many of Green's earlier papers were published in international specialist journals, in subsequent years his papers did not attract the same audience and largely appeared in the *New Zealand Medical Journal*.

Green was not an unintelligent man, and by the mid-1970s he had witnessed many women in his study developing cancer, so one must assume he knew his experiment had failed. Liam Wright, who worked with Green on the cervical cancer team for many years and had seen and treated many of Green's CIS patients who had progressed to cervical cancer, told me Green had later admitted to him that 'some cases might progress'.[26]

When a group of Waikato colleagues offered to write a letter supportive of Green to the *New Zealand Herald* stating that, while they did not currently follow his management of CIS, they did concede his earlier, non-hysterectomy approach had been entirely motivated for the welfare of women, Green responded, 'Don't write your letter; I'm going down and I don't want to contaminate you.'[27] When Dr Louis Schellekens, from the Netherlands, visited NWH on the day Green retired in 1982, he told Green he had read his papers and did not agree CIS was harmless. Green responded, 'Did you believe that nonsense? Carcinoma *in-situ* is dangerous, so take it out, remove it.'[28]

CHAPTER 14

MEA CULPA

Bill Liley and I both understood about scientific research and hypotheses at
that time but chose not to intervene but to turn a blind eye.

MONT LIGGINS

COULD ANYONE HAVE DISSUADED Green from persisting with his
experiment? Most unlikely, although in my view there is one possible
candidate – Professor (later Sir) Mont Liggins. He was unquestionably New
Zealand's finest mind at the time in obstetrics and gynaecology, and a world
leader in perinatal research; his many honours attest to this. In 1976 I was
privileged to join C Team as a visiting consultant under Liggins' leadership
and I remain grateful for his teaching. I was both in awe of, and somewhat
intimidated by, the rigorous scientific intellect he applied to clinical
medicine; on occasions he demonstrated a whiff of intellectual superiority.

Liggins' research centred on pre-term labour. In an age when induction
of labour had become commonplace, under his influence it was very
uncommon – wherever possible, labour was to be a natural, spontaneous
event. Understandably, in late pregnancy, patients and doctors in high-risk
situations became extremely anxious as they waited for a precious baby
to arrive. Not infrequently the slightest niggle was sufficient to hasten a
woman to the delivery ward to expedite the birth – while Liggins slept.

Surprisingly, Liggins, who had not previously demonstrated any
interest in cervical precancer or cancer, attended a meeting at the Auckland
Medical School on the subject a short time after the publication of our
1984 paper (which we knew had been discussed in the department) and
made disparaging comments on the role of colposcopy. The following year,
and shortly before the *Metro* article was published, he co-authored, with
Bonham and Green, a deprecatory article in the *Australia and New Zealand
Journal of Obstetrics and Gynaecology*, questioning the value of cervical
screening, its 'economic sense' and the 'huge capital investment' it would
require, and making a plea for future studies of the natural history of CIS of

the cervix.[1] They ignored the overwhelming epidemiological evidence, and the new evidence that the human papilloma virus (HPV) was the central causative factor in cervical cancer. They also ignored the findings of our 1984 paper from their own hospital.

If Liggins supported Green, why didn't he accede to the pleas from Green's wife, Joan, to come forward and provide defence for him in the witness box at the Cartwright Inquiry? Despite my contention that Green could have discussed his experiment with Liggins, Liley and other professional friends, a friend and colleague of all three men has noted: 'Over the years, talking at National Women's Hospital with Mont, Herb and Bill, there was never reference to Herb's [academic] interests and I wonder now how they were never discussed to advantage among themselves.'[2] The answer is simple: none of us likes to confront friends who have strongly held opinions that are contrary to our own – especially if we fear their reaction.

Much later Barbara Heslop articulated what many were thinking at the time: 'Where were Mont Liggins and the others? He was a friend of Herb's and was going to be asked at the Inquiry if Herb's [experiment] was research. Technically it was, and he didn't want to say so and thereby to stab his friend in the back, so he contrived to be out of the country.'[3]

In 2004 Heslop published a paper entitled 'All about research: Looking back at the 1987 Cervical Cancer Inquiry'.[4] Soon after, I contacted her, then visited her on a number of occasions and began a correspondence that lasted until her death. She was a medical school classmate of Liggins, had an equally fine intellect and, importantly, because she worked in Dunedin, was removed from the local loyalties of Auckland. Heslop later gave me the correspondence she had had with Liggins around the time she published her paper. Aware that I was writing this book, of which she read a draft, she wanted me to have them in order that 'the truth isn't lost'. Liggins had had plenty of time to reflect on the whole episode. He wrote to her:

The fatal flaw to Herb's approach was that he never saw it as an experiment but as simply a follow-up study of a particular treatment – like following up 1000 appendectomies to see how many patients died or had complications like a peritonitis, bowel obstruction and so on. That it was an experiment with two possible endpoints – invasive cancer or no invasive cancer – did not occur to him ... Herb being Herb knew that he was right and there would be no invasive cancer.

For many years, Liggins continued, it seemed that Green was correct. 'The incidence of cancer in this group was no higher than the expected ... mainly because of the long, latent period to progression to cancer, but also because he was in the habit of reviewing Jock McLean's pathology diagnoses. ... You can imagine how Jock felt about that. Although Herb and Bill McIndoe had a bitter falling-out at a later date, for a long time Herb was only too happy to accept his colposcopy follow-up.' Liggins also pointed out that an

> unbiased peer review [of Green's study] would have been impossible to get. I don't think there was a peer in the world who would not relish the opportunity to put a knife in Herb's back even though none of them had any better evidence of whether carcinoma in-situ was or was not a precursor. In fact Herb's study remains the solidest evidence that progression [of carcinoma in-situ] does occur. He certainly did not plan it that way. Had he done so, with death from invasive cancer as an endpoint, it would not have got approval from the ethics committee [i.e. the Hospital Medical Committee]. I have borne a burden of guilt for not having seen the study for what it was at the outset. We were close friends, and partners in a forestry venture and I admired his clinical skills and his empathy for his patients, foreign students and the underdog in general. Seeing the truth with so much baggage aboard was not easy.

Three months later Liggins again wrote to Heslop to say that in 'All about research' she had 'got it right and I would not want you to change any of it. It shows a remarkably accurate understanding of the research climate of the time. It also renews my feeling of guilt about the whole affair. Bill Liley and I both understood about scientific research and hypotheses at that time but we chose not to try to intervene but to turn a blind eye.'

Liggins was not alone; everyone turned a blind eye. This was a systemic failure.

Liggins explained that he was 'in a difficult position' during the inquiry:

> I was expected to advise Herb's lawyer because by then, with the benefit of hindsight, I had to agree with Jim Hodge [Medical Research Council Director] that it was an experiment ... I must have had some reservations early on because on occasions when Herb was overseas my wife and I took the opportunity of doing a hysterectomy on patients with persistent positive smears and risking Herb's wrath when he returned.[5]

These were remarkable admissions. Liggins and Liley, the men responsible for saving the lives of countless premature babies, put loyalty to their old friend and colleague ahead of their concerns for the women in Green's experiment. Around the time of the 1975 working party inquiry and report, McIndoe approached Liggins seeking his advice on how to deal with the consequences of Green's experiment. Liggins strongly defended Green, asking McIndoe, 'Are you questioning his veracity?' McIndoe responded immediately, 'That is the question.'[6]

By the time of the inquiry it was too late; Liggins' moral courage continued to fail him and he avoided the witness box. A widely circulated, off-the-cuff comment by Green's lawyer, David Collins, was that his only success at the inquiry was keeping Mont Liggins out of the witness box.[7] Whether that comment was made by Collins, and whether or not it is a fair appraisal, its circulation is a clear indication of the significance of Liggins' absence from the hearings.

By the time Liggins wrote these mea culpas in 2004 he was a knight of the realm, a Fellow of the Royal Society (of London) and a national icon. His preceding silence not only maintained his scientific reputation, but also served to sustain Bonham's silence and that of the other members of the senior academic and clinical staff in their continuing denial.

In a letter to me, Heslop observed that Liggins

was in a no-win situation in respect to the inquiry. He couldn't give an honest, scientific opinion of Herb's project without inflicting substantial damage on his friends and National Women's colleagues, on himself for not having intervened earlier, and also on Herb's legal defence which was based on the 'partial treatment' argument. An honest opinion would have been a very public knife in the back for Herb. I suspect that he just couldn't do it. There was little doubt that Herb's project was research by any definition.[8]

Professor Mark Henaghan has observed that the 'unfortunate experiment' was the catalyst in undermining trust between New Zealand doctors and their patients.[9] This is only partly true. By the time of the Cartwright Inquiry in 1987, patients (and journalists) were already beginning to ask hard questions. It should not be forgotten that two decades earlier, when Green was questioning scientific doctrine, many other sacred truths were being challenged, in protests over civil rights, the role of women, war and peace, the authority of the church ... It was an era of great change. Visiting British academic Klim McPherson pointed out shortly after the inquiry was over and the report out, 'Trust cannot be fully restored unless and until organised medicine in New Zealand stands up and can be clearly seen to regret and to be responding to what has unambiguously happened.'[10] And trust, wrote distinguished New Zealand academic Annette Baier, 'is appropriately placed in those who, for whatever motives, welcome the equalisation of power, who assist the less powerful and renounce eminence of power.'[11]

In the view of Professor Charlotte Paul, 'in the end it was McIndoe and McLean's personal morality that counted'. Their actions in objecting to Green's experiment, and in writing up the results, were models of good practice in medicine. However, once the Cartwright Report came out, 'The leaders of the medical profession in 1988 did not acknowledge publicly, either that patients had been harmed, or the profession's responsibility in failing to stop Green. They also never identified nor praised the whistle-blowers.'[12] For Paul the main power problem lay within the profession: 'The crucial problem of power which led to failure to stop the trial was the imbalance of power among doctors. There was extreme difficulty in challenging the powerful medical leaders in the hospital, with rigid hierarchies and strong personalities.'[13]

Changing moral values, which were not within the ambit of the commission of inquiry – are understandably problematic. Cartwright touched on the central moral themes when she observed that the in-house working party 'avoided the real issues'. The central moral themes of this story – turning a blind eye and misplaced loyalty – remain with us and continue to surface.

It is easy for us today to sit in judgement on Bonham, Liggins and many of the other members of the NWH senior staff. We have all been guilty of misplaced loyalty; we have all turned a blind eye; we are all human. McIndoe and McLean themselves exhibited human failings, but at least these men at the bottom of the medical hierarchy were advocates for the patients first.

It is inappropriate to draw comparisons between the unfortunate experiment and the Jewish holocaust, as some have done.[14] Nonetheless, parallels can be drawn between the behaviour of some German scientists, including a number of Nobel Prize winners, around the time of World War II, and the events at NWH in relation to the moral responsibilities of practitioners. In his book *Serving the Reich*, Philip Ball wrote: 'There are a few heroes and villains in this tale. But most of the players are, like most of us, neither of these things. Their flaws, misjudgements, their kindnesses and acts of bravery, are ours: compromised and myopic, perhaps, beyond good and evil – and human, all too human.'[15]

Mike Taylor has noted, 'The fundamental strength of science is to force its practitioners to confront their own fallibility.' And he suggests that 'the core, immutable quality of science' is humility:

> Everyone knows it's good to be able to admit when we've been wrong about something. We all like to see that quality in others. We all like to think that we possess it ourselves – although, needless to say, in our case it never comes up, because we don't make mistakes. And there's the rub. It goes very, very strongly against the grain for us to admit the possibility of error in our own work …
>
> But science that we can build on needs to be right. That means that when we're wrong – and we will be from time to time, unless we're doing terribly unambitious work – our wrong results need to be corrected.
>
> It's because we're not humble by nature – because we need to have humility formally imposed on us …[16]

One evening late in 1990 Bernie Kyle, a contemporary of Green and a man who possessed one of the finest minds in the hospital, discussed with me the background to Green's failed experiment. The following day he set out his views in writing. He began by stressing that 1966, when the meeting was held to discuss allowing Green to carry out his study, was 'a time when ethical considerations did not assume the importance they did ten or more years later'. The matter was fully discussed and the ensuing decision was not hasty. 'It is quite wrong to consider and judge the matter in the light of 1990 knowledge.' Kyle continued:

> we trusted people, colleagues, to behave ethically and I don't think it entered the heads of any of the members of the HMC [the Hospital Medical Committee and the Senior Medical Staff] that those engaged in so-called research would act otherwise. Events later proved us wrong and this came as a painful shock. Nobody at the time would have believed any of their colleagues would have 'cooked' the results. There was old-fashioned trust, if you like, and we naively took people at their word. How false this was.

There were, he noted, 'inbuilt safeguards in the project ... The most compelling of these was if anyone expressed doubt about any aspect of the project then it would be stopped and the matter looked into.' In his words Green 'just blundered on with disregard for everyone, especially those so vitally concerned, the patients – the unwitting subjects of this so-called piece of research. I don't think anyone on the HMC would have thought they would be so treacherously betrayed. Such conduct was not known at that time. The go ahead was given in good faith.'

In considering why the project was not stopped as soon as it was discovered to be flawed, Kyle thought there were several explanations: 'a laissez-faire attitude' by the committee members, most of whom wanted to keep on side with the university; 'disbelief anything untoward would be happening in a research project in the hospital' (especially a university project); and 'the fundamental fact that members ... were entrenched in the committee and did not want anything to "rock the boat"'. In Kyle's opinion, the composition of the committees, and the way they had originally been set up, contributed to 'the recipe for trouble and disaster which had yet to come ... and was always to be a cause of contention'. Then there was the 'arrogance of some of the university staff, two in particular'.[17]

***

Standing back after more than 30 years I can recognise two quite separate chapters in the story of the 'unfortunate experiment'. The first, between 1966 and 1987, was the struggle between the little men at the bottom of the medical hierarchy at NWH and the powerful academic unit, which seemingly demonstrated no empathy for the increasing number of women victims. The second phase, after the inquiry in 1987, was the conflict between a powerful, determined and well-organised feminist lobby and a poorly prepared and disorganised group of senior doctors who continued to maintain a 'defend and deny' stance. But the victims were at last being heard.

Late in life Green wrote a long letter with marked religious overtones to his old physician colleague, Dr Basil Quin. He was clearly depressed but felt God would be his judge and history would vindicate him.[18] It is interesting that many of those closest to this tragedy have admitted to the truth in late-life mea culpas, while some with more tenuous connections continue to defend Green's actions.

The ongoing debate, the revisionism – and this book – could have been avoided had more of the profession faced up to the outcome of the experiment and the findings of the subsequent inquiry. The medical profession rightly prides itself on being a 'caring' community. Sadly, in this story, a small group of powerful senior doctors placed their profession before their patients. This generally defensive approach taken by so many has given the impression that the impetus for change and improvement is reactive, not proactive. This story will end only when there has been an unqualified acceptance that there was an experiment that resulted in unnecessary suffering and death, and an unqualified apology. It can have no ending while denial exists. The obdurate and continuing refusal of influential sections of the medical profession to acknowledge the experiment and its consequences has served only to prolong divisions within the profession and the community.

I am deeply sorry for what happened to Bonham and Green, but my thoughts are with the hundreds of women and their families who were unknowing actors in Green's experiment. Some were lucky, as the CIS lesion disappeared spontaneously following their diagnostic biopsies; some were fortunate to then go on and bear children; some were able to remove themselves from Green's clinic and, at some personal cost, have private treatment that eradicated the disease. But there were many who suffered significantly as a result of the multiple biopsies performed over the years, which for some resulted in sterility, and in others led to hysterectomy. Some, like 'Ruth', were discharged from Green's care with scarred cervices, preventing the future taking of accurate smears, having been assured they were not at increased risk of developing cancer – only to return with it later. Many unfortunate women, after years and years of abnormal smears, developed cancer, resulting in a total disruption of their lives and those of their families; some died. We must never forget these women.

I concede that Green was a man from an earlier age, a time when the science of clinical medicine was less developed and ethical codes were new. His motives were entirely transparent – he made no secret of his experiment. I cannot extend my generosity to the modern generation of academic revisionists who hide behind a smokescreen of semantics, who interview books and not people, and who misrepresent the evidence and blame others for Green's downfall. Their claims – in favour of Green's approach to his patients, and his conclusions – and their criticisms of those of us who uncovered the flaws in his study, are specious and dishonest.

The 1964 Declaration of Helsinki, developed by the World Medical Association 'as a statement of ethical principles for medical research involving human subjects, including research on identifiable human material and data',[19] states: 'The doctor can combine clinical research with professional care, the object being the acquisition of new knowledge, only to the extent that clinical research is justified by the therapeutic value for the patient.'[20]

A quarter of a century ago the NWH Medical Committee rescinded an apology to the women affected by the experiment. There is still no apology. Neither has there been an apology from the New Zealand Council of the Royal Australian and New Zealand College of Obstetricians and Gynaecologists. Following the Cartwright Inquiry the dean of the Auckland Medical School said, in a television interview, that the university had wanted to apologise to the women damaged by the 'unfortunate experiment' but their lawyers had advised them not to.[21] Belatedly he himself did apologise. It is my hope that some time in the future a new generation of obstetricians and gynaecologists will see fit to acknowledge the wrong, and say they are sorry.

EPILOGUE

*He [Green] so believed he was right he was not seeing the
results of what he was doing.*

Dennis Bonham

Soon after Bonham had been censured and found guilty of
disgraceful conduct by the Medical Council, he spoke to the *Sunday
Star*. Under the headline, 'It was wrong, says Bonham', he said he was
understandably disappointed by the inquiry's outcome. Nonetheless his
responses were refreshingly honest. He admitted he 'and Green certainly
held different views' on a range of issues, describing Green's approach as
being 'so conservative that it bordered on fanaticism … his enthusiasm for
conservatism led him to under-treat patients. He so believed he was right he
was not seeing the results of what he was doing.' Bonham admitted that he
should 'have distanced himself from Green's approach'. He also noted that
Green was a 'soloist like most of my staff were. People who do fairly brilliant
things tend to be soloists and not too much part of a team.' He claimed that
if he was culpable, so were all the senior gynaecological staff at NWH, and
he finally conceded that 'there was a weakness in my administration'.[1]

Bonham and I became progressively estranged after I delivered him a
pre-publication copy of the 1984 paper. Some years after his retirement in
1986 I decided to visit him. Acting on an impulse, I phoned the Bonham
home and told a surprised Nancie I would like to visit Dennis; she graciously
invited me to afternoon tea.

In the years since his retirement Dennis, the former colossus, had
become a frail old man. He welcomed me warmly. When I explained that I
wished to thank him for his contributions to medical education and to the
health of New Zealand women and children, tears came to his eyes. Nancie
served tea as we moved to common ground – the debacles occurring in the
'new' hospital management system.

His frailty brought home to me the frailty of all of us involved in this sad affair. To Bonham's credit, he did finally accept that misguided loyalty had influenced his actions, but it was too late – his and Green's careers were in tatters. Green never recanted.

REVISIONISM AND DENIAL

The current reaction of the medical profession does not bode well.
The mode is denial.

SANDRA CONEY

ON VALENTINE'S DAY 2014 a meeting was held to celebrate the 50th anniversary of the opening of the second (1964) NWH building. The programme was carefully scripted by Tony Baird, president of the New Zealand Medical Association, who chaired the gathering. The event revealed still visible scars; not all participants in the story had yet conveniently faded away.

One of those in attendance that day was Linda Bryder, who, three years before, when associate professor of history at Auckland University, had written a controversial book, *A History of the 'Unfortunate Experiment' at National Women's Hospital*, which had been promoted at the NWH Senior Medical Officers' meeting.[1] In this she argued, to use the words of Joanna Manning, associate professor of law at the same university, that:

> there was no experiment; that Green's patients merely received 'conservative' treatment; that Green was not the maverick he was made out to be, but rather was one of a number of 'thinking gynaecologists' who advocated a similar approach as being safe; that Green and his colleagues were far from being alone in the world in questioning the benefits of population-based cervical screening; that the patients were adequately informed according to current standards; and that patients were unharmed as Green followed them assiduously, not just in the interests of science, but to ensure their safety and well-being.[2]

As Manning pointed out, because the Cartwright Inquiry dealt with critical issues – 'matters of life and death for the patients; the professional reputations of Coney and Bunkle; the life's work and professional reputations of leaders within the medical profession; and, to a significant extent, public trust and confidence in the profession, and its own sense of self-worth' – its findings were likely to be challenged. But, in her view, 'Bryder's interpretation of the inquiry, like Corbett's [*Metro*'s "Second thoughts" article], is essentially political, emphasising Coney and Bunkle's "feminist agenda" of breaking the power of the medical profession, [a power] which [they] saw as damaging to women.'[3]

Bryder's book also received strong criticism from fellow medical historian Professor Barbara Brookes of the University of Otago. Historians, Brookes wrote, have a responsibility 'to weigh and respect their sources, and quote them accurately; to seek all relevant sources to gain a multi-faceted view; and to interpret the past in a coherent and judicious way ... Failure to seek expert opinion from various sides of a question raises doubts about whether the historian's approach is sufficiently judicious.' Brookes found it 'most surprising' that Bryder did not seek to interview some of the key players, including Hugh Rennie and David Skegg – 'and in particular Ron Jones, who worked with Green at National Women's and is the only surviving gynaecologist author of the important 1984 paper which exposed the dangers of Green's practice. Had she questioned Jones about the paper and its intent, many of her concerns about misinterpretation might well have been resolved.'[4]

Professor Charlotte Paul believed that Bryder's 'misrepresentation of the medical context should be of serious concern to the profession in New Zealand'. Patients and their needs should be put first, and high standards of scientific conduct adhered to. 'If this distorted story of blameless doctors, grateful patients, and normal scientific conduct is accepted it will set back the profession's difficult task of acknowledging and trying to learn from error.'[5] Paul also noted that Bryder appeared to have based her work on 'an interpretation of events by a number of gynaecologists who remained loyal to Green and [were] aggrieved about the Inquiry'.[6]

The title of this book, *Doctors in Denial*, refers not only to the doctors of National Women's Hospital at the time who failed to act through apathy, detachment or misplaced loyalty, but also to those today who, ignoring the suffering of many women in Green's experiment, have embraced the revisionism that I believe is integral to Bryder's book. The wilful blindness of some of the younger generation of doctors is inexcusable. These well-educated younger men and women cannot be forgiven for failing to understand the science, the ethics and the disastrous consequences for the women involved in Green's experiment. Their failing is one of uncritical and misplaced loyalty to old teachers. A younger colleague returning to practise in New Zealand some years after the inquiry told me in all seriousness, 'Bloody Cartwright has fucked up my whole career.'

When Dan O'Connor presented a talk on the 'unfortunate experiment' at a medico-legal dinner in Brisbane in 1991, he was

> hounded by a group of New Zealand doctors who attended the dinner specifically to get stuck into me for daring to mention Herb Green's name in public. His disciples have a uniquely blind faith which quite surprises me. A psychiatrist delivered not only a eulogy on behalf of Herb at the end of my paper, but a vicious attack on McIndoe and McLean. A truly sad era in medical history for all of us and especially so, I suspect, for those of you who are involved at the coalface.[7]

The immense disparity between Professor Bryder's perception of the unfortunate experiment and that of David Skegg, a distinguished authority in the field of cancer epidemiology, was illustrated in a September 2009 story in the *New Zealand Herald* under the headline 'An unfortunate fallout: Academics against revisionist history'. Skegg observed, 'I assume Professor Bryder misunderstands the scientific evidence about Green's study because otherwise she would be guilty of deliberate obfuscation.' Bryder in her response dismissed this comment: 'I do not see how interviewing Professor Skegg about the 1984 paper would have added anything to [my] understanding of its content.'[8]

The acrimonious debate that followed the publication of Bryder's book illustrates the ongoing deep division between those who continue to defend and deny the damage caused by the experiment and those of us who have acknowledged it. The dispute will persist until there is universal acknowledgement of what Green did and the harm it caused.

Perhaps there will always be people who try to rationalise unethical behaviour for their own ends. Paul and Brookes picked up this theme and have compared the way Bryder and her sympathisers have rationalised Green's research with those who defended the investigators in the Tuskegee Study. They describe scientific, political and moral rationalisations that have been used by defenders of both studies. Politics were in play in the studies' coming to public notice. But, contrary to the defenders, those who brought the studies to public attention did not misread the evidence. Instead they opened up the debate, which allowed the wider public to know what had happened and to see the exploitation with fresh eyes.[9]

* * *

This book began at meetings in London, and in Auckland, held with the purpose of selecting New Zealand's next postgraduate professor of obstetrics and gynaecology. It ends in the mediaeval colleges of Oxford and Cambridge universities.

At the anniversary meeting in February 2014 Linda Bryder invited a mentor, Professor Sir Iain Chalmers, to speak to the audience via a video link from Oxford University. Chalmers had for many years headed the Cochrane Collaboration, which aimed to produce evidence-based guidelines to assist doctors in providing the best management of medical conditions. He began by praising the quality of Liggins' research, then went on to criticise the 'investigative quality of the Cartwright Inquiry' and warn of the 'dire consequences of ignoring research evidence'.

This was extraordinary. A New Zealand historian, possibly in liaison with some NWH gynaecologists, suggesting to a semi-retired Oxford professor that he speak to the shortcomings of the Cartwright Inquiry, at a celebratory event for the hospital some 26 years later.[10] His presentation defended Green's experiment and ignored the harm arising from it. Chalmers' words shocked many of us in the audience. That evening, on national television, Linda Bryder said that Green's approach was 'not experimental in the same way they [McIndoe, McLean and Jones] claimed; it was indeed practised by many of the more progressive gynaecologists around the world'.[11] This is simply not true: gynaecologists elsewhere sought to eradicate the lesion, not observe it.

I subsequently wrote to Chalmers, and asked him the same question I had previously asked Bryder: 'Why did so many women develop cancer?'[12] Like Bryder, he steadfastly refused to answer my question, arguing instead that Green avoided 'morbidity, unwanted infertility and possible death resulting from the complications of over-treatment' of CIS. I have never encountered a death from the treatment of CIS but I have seen women with untreated CIS develop cancer and die. CIS is at the most severe end of the spectrum of pre-cancerous changes; there is no buffer zone before invasive cancer. As Liggins said, 'There is either cancer or no cancer'.[13] Invite any woman to make a choice between a 30–50 per cent chance of developing cancer from untreated or inadequately treated CIS, and the 'complications of over-treatment'[14] Chalmers claimed, and I know what most women would choose.

In 2010 I was a co-author of a paper that described Green's patients being managed according to Chalmers' definition of Green's 'repeated observation without initial intervention'. The group of women studied in this paper had a 10 times greater risk of developing cancer than women treated with curative intent.[15] Almost all deaths were in this group.

During the course of his presentation, Chalmers referred to a review of Bryder's book by a retired New Zealand medical researcher, Professor Robin Carrell, who studied blood disorders while at Cambridge University. Carrell claimed Bryder had 'put the record straight' and 'the inquiry [was] a trial by media' led by 'an aggressive advocate for the feminists'.[16] The inquiry was not about feminism, nor was it a 'trial by media' – it was an investigation into an unethical experiment on women, ending for some in cancer and death. Feminism was, however, the catalyst that brought the unethical experiment to the attention of the public. Feminists remain convenient scapegoats for those who continue to criticise the Cartwright Inquiry. As Ellie May O'Hagan has pointed out, 'popular, non-threatening feminism is destined for failure … it's anger that changes the world.'[17] New Zealand women should be grateful that angry feminists challenged the academic hierarchy at NWH. It is disappointing that even after all these years a highly placed coterie of individuals continues to deny Green's experiment and its appalling consequences.

SUMMARY OF MAIN FINDINGS OF THE CARTWRIGHT INQUIRY

1. There was a failure to treat cervical carcinoma in situ (CIS) adequately at National Women's Hospital.

(a) The outcome of treatment for the majority of women has been adequate, although a significant number were not managed by generally accepted standards over a period of years. For a minority of women, management resulted in persisting disease, the development of invasive cancer and, in some cases, death.

(b) The reasons for the failure were:

- the implementation of the procedures advocated in the 1966 trial;
- failure to recognise the dangers for patients in departing from accepted standards of treatment;
- failure to evaluate the risks to patients if the hypothesis on which the trial was based was incorrect;
- failure to note the rising incidence of invasive cancer and to stop the trial and treat the patients as soon as cogent evidence of risk began to emerge;
- failure of some colleagues and the administration to act decisively in the interests of patients' safety.

2. A research programme into the natural history of CIS of the genital tract was conducted at National Women's Hospital.

(a) There was one major trial (the 1966 trial) into the natural history of CIS, and some supplementary research, involving vaginal swabs of newborn female infants and a study of the histology of fetal cervices from aborted and stillborn infants.

(b) The great majority of patients did not know, except intuitively, that they were participants in the 1966 trial. No formal consent was sought from the parents of 2244 newborn babies who were swabbed, or from parents for the study of fetal cervices.

(c) From 1966 to 1987 there were many and varied expressions of concern about the 1966 trial, both from within New Zealand and overseas. The trial was reviewed by the Hospital Medical Committee in 1975, but not formally ended.

3. Further advice or treatment, or both, should be offered to women who have been under the care of National Women's Hospital with CIS, where there was doubt about the adequacy of their treatment. This includes 20 patients with persistent or recurrent abnormal cytology; 13 patients with a diagnosis of microinvasive carcinoma; 13 patients whose last operative procedure showed incomplete excision; and 5 patients who have never had more than a punch or wedge biopsy.

ENDNOTES

INTRODUCTION

1. S. Cartwright, *The Report of the Committee of Inquiry into Allegations Concerning the Treatment of Cervical Cancer at National Women's Hospital and into Other Related Matters* (Auckland: Government Printing Office, 1988); S. Coney, *The Unfortunate Experiment: The full story behind the inquiry into cervical cancer treatment* (Auckland: Penguin Books, 1998).

2. M.R. McCredie, C. Paul, K. Sharples, J. Baranyai, G. Medley, D.C. Skegg & R.W. Jones, 'Consequences in participating in a study of the natural history of cervical intraepithelial neoplasia 3', *Australia and New Zealand Journal of Obstetrics and Gynaecology* 50, 2010, 363–70; M.R. McCredie, K. Sharples, C. Paul, J. Baranyai, G. Medley, D.C. Skegg & R.W. Jones, 'Natural history of cervical neoplasia and risk of invasive cancer in women with cervical intraepithelial neoplasia 3: A retrospective cohort study', *Lancet Oncology* 9, 2008, 425–34.

CHAPTER 1: A PROFESSORIAL APPOINTMENT

1. N.R. Butler, D.G. Bonham, *Perinatal Mortality: The first report of the 1958 British Perinatal Mortality Survey under the auspices of National Birthday Trust Fund* (London: E. & S. Livingstone, 1963); A.W. Liley, 'Intrauterine transfusion of fetus in haemolytic disease', *British Medical Journal* 5365, 2 November 1963, 1107–09; G.C. Liggins & R.N. Howie, 'A controlled trial of antepartum glucocorticoid treatment for prevention of respiratory distress syndrome in premature infants', *Paediatrics* 50, 1972, 515–25.

2. G.H. Green, 'Cervical carcinoma *in-situ*: An atypical viewpoint', *Australia and New Zealand Journal of Obstetrics and Gynaecology* 10, 1970, 41–48; 'Forum: Has the survival rate from invasive carcinoma of the cervix been influenced by cervical screening?', *Modern Medicine USA*, 20 September 1971, 180–88; G.H. Green, 'Cervical cancer and cytology screening in New Zealand', *British Journal of Obstetrics and Gynaecology* 85, 1978, 881–86; G. Johannesson & N.E. Day, Correspondence, *British Journal of Obstetrics and Gynaecology* 86, 1979, 671–72.

3. G. Wakely, 'For the women of New Zealand: The story of the National Women's Hospital' (unpublished, 1963), R.W. Jones, personal papers; Minutes of the New Zealand Obstetric and Gynaecological Society, vol. 1, 11 December 1940, 196.

4. Ibid.

5. G.H. Green, chapter on the history of the Postgraduate School of Obstetrics and Gynaecology, in H.D. Erlam (ed.), *A Notable Result: An historical essay on the beginnings and first fifteen years of the School of Medicine* (Auckland: University of Auckland School of Medicine, 1983), 68.
6. University of Auckland Council Papers, 1963.
7. Obituary, B.V. Kyle, *New Zealand Medical Journal* 121, 2008, 1269.
8. G. Chamberlain, *Special Delivery: The life of the celebrated British obstetrician William Nixon* (London: Royal College of Obstetricians and Gynaecologists Press, 2004), 87–94.
9. Ibid.
10. H.C. McLaren, M.E. Attwood, W.C. Nixon, D.G. Bonham, D.J. MacRae, D.F. Hawkins & B. Eton, 'Discussion on the cervix–antepartum and postpartum', *Proceedings of the Royal Society of Medicine* 54, 1961, 712–20.
11. D.G. Bonham & D.F. Gibb, 'A new enzyme test for gynaecological cancer', *British Medical Journal* 2 (5308), 1962, 823–44.
12. M.J. Churchouse, G.N. Carter & D.G. Bonham, 'The source of 6-phosphogluconate dehydrogenase in vaginal fluid samples', *Journal of Obstetrics and Gynaecology of the British Commonwealth* 74, 1967, 712–22.
13. D.F. Hawkins, communication with the author, 16 September 2005.
14. D.G. Bonham, in *Family Planning Association Journal*, 1964. Quoted by Green in undated notes given to students to emphasise his point of view.
15. G.H. Green, 'Quotations for students', R.W. Jones papers.
16. D. Cole, communication with the author, 15 January 2008.
17. J. Gudex, communication with the author, 9 August 2012.
18. G.H. Green, Transcript of Public Hearings to the Committee of Inquiry into Allegations Concerning the Treatment of Cervical Cancer at National Women's Hospital and into Other Related Matters, Archives New Zealand BAGC 18494 A638/186/a.
19. B.F. Heslop, communication with the author, 28 October 2007.
20. P. Warren, communication with the author, 2005. Dr Tony Crick was the brother of Francis Crick who, with James Watson and New Zealand-born Maurice Wilkins, was awarded the 1962 Nobel Prize in Physiology or Medicine for the discovery of the structure of DNA.
21. B.V. Kyle, communication with the author, 1990.
22. R. Gudex, communication with the author, 3 August 2012.
23. J. Finlay, communication with the author, 2005.
24. J.H. Taylor, communication with the author, 1992.
25. M. Falloon, communication with the author, 1988.
26. Green, Transcript of Public Hearings to the Committee of Inquiry …, Archives New Zealand BAGC 18494 A638/186/a.

27. University of Auckland Council papers, 1963.
28. D. Robb, *Medical Odyssey* (Auckland: Collins, 1967).
29. Obituary, D. Robb, *New Zealand Medical Journal* 80, 1974, 128–32.
30. Ibid.
31. University of Auckland Council papers, 1963.
32. G.H. Green, 'Letter from New Zealand: New York horizons', *Bulletin of the Sloane Hospital for Women* 9, Winter 1963, 133–36.
33. D. Menzies, communication with the author, 12 October 2005.
34. J. Harbutt, communication with the author, 14 February 1995.
35. University of Auckland Council papers, 1963.
36. Adequacy of Medical Statistics in New Zealand, report of ad hoc committee of Medical Research Council of New Zealand, chaired by G.H. Green, November 1969.
37. M. Sparrow, *Abortion Then and Now* (Wellington: Victoria University Press, 2010).
38. G.H. Green, 'Tubal ligation', *New Zealand Medical Journal* 57, 1958, 470–77.
39. Green, Transcript of Public Hearings to the Committee of Inquiry …, Archives New Zealand BAGC 18494 A638/186/a.
40. G.H. Green, correspondence with J.R. Dobson, 25 June 1975. In the author's possession.
41. Sparrow, *Abortion Then and Now*.
42. J. Werry, communication with the author, 1 February 2012.
43. G.H. Green, *Introduction to Obstetrics* (Christchurch: N.M. Peryer, 4 edns, 1962–82); R. Gudex, communication with the author, 3 August 2012.
44. R. Jackson, communication with the author, 2011.
45. G.H. Green, 'A Tudor caesarean section', *Surgery, Gynecology and Obstetrics* 161, 1985, 490–96; G.H. Green, 'A royal obstetric tragedy and the epitaph', *NZ Nursing Journal*, July 1969, 7–11.
46. J. Dewhurst, communication with the author, 23 November 2004.
47. Ibid.
48. M. Belgrave, *The Mater: A history of Auckland's Mercy Hospital 1900–2000* (Auckland: Mercy Hospital, 2000), 171–72.
49. R.W. Jones papers.
50. Obituary, D.G. Bonham, *University of Auckland News* 35, 2005, 20–21.
51. Ibid.
52. D.F. Hawkins, communication with the author, 16 September 2005; D. Menzies, communication with the author, 12 October 2005.
53. Obituary, D.G. Bonham.
54. J. Werry, communication with the author, 1 February 2012.
55. J. McDonald, communication with the author, 2012.

56. J. Carnachan, communication with the author, 2012.
57. C. Hoskins, communication with the author, 2009.
58. J. Carnachan, communication with the author, 2012.
59. R.W. Jones papers.
60. National Health Statistics Centre, 'Perinatal mortality in New Zealand 1972–73', Special Report Series 50 (Wellington: Department of Health, 1977); R.N. Howie, 'Credit where credit's due', *New Zealand Herald*, 20 July 2005.
61. J.D. Kim, communication with the author, 22 December 2005.
62. P. Nash, communication with the author, 2014.
63. M. Churchouse, 'The Greening of cytology' (unpublished), 25 May 2010. In the author's possession.
64. R. Jackson, communication with the author, 2011.
65. I. Asher, communication with the author, 9 October 2012.
66. G.H. Green, 'Cervical cancer and cytology screening', *Modern Medicine of New Zealand*, 16 August 1976, 46.
67. 'DES not the villain, says doctor', *Auckland Star*, 28 August 1981.
68. R. Doll, 'Concluding remarks', Medical Research Council Epidemiology Symposium, Auckland, 2 November 1973, *New Zealand Medical Journal* 80, 1974, 403–04.
69. L. Wright, communication with the author, 23 October 2001.
70. G.C. Liggins, *University of Auckland News* 11, 1981, 31.
71. J. Werry, communication with the author, 1 February 2012.
72. H. Doerr, communication with the author, 2012.
73. I. Fisher communication with the author, 28 February 2005.
74. D.G. Bonham, Affidavit to Medical Council, 1990, 22.

CHAPTER 2: THE EVOLUTION OF A DISBELIEF ...

1. J. Williams, Harveian Lectures for 1886: 'On cancer of the uterus', *Lancet*, 1 January 1887, 6–9; 8 January 1887, 59–62.
2. Verdalle, 1903, cited in O. Petersen, 'Precancerous changes in the cervical epithelium in relation to manifest cervical cancer', *Acta Radiologica*, supplement 127, 1955.
3. W. Schauenstein, 1908, cited in O. Petersen, 'Precancerous changes ...'; I.C. Rubin, 'The pathological diagnosis of incipient carcinoma of the uterus', *American Journal of Obstetrics and Diseases of Women and Children* 62, 1910, 668–76.
4. A.C. Broders, 'Carcinoma *in-situ* contrasted with benign penetrating epithelium', *Journal of the American Medical Association* 99, 1932, 1670–74.
5. J.W. Reagan, I.L. Seidemann & Y. Saracusa, 'The cellular morphology of carcinoma *in-situ* and dysplasia or atypical hyperplasia of the uterine cervix', *Cancer* 6, 1953, 224–35.

6. R.M. Richart, 'Influence of diagnostic and therapeutic procedures on the distribution of cervical intraepithelial neoplasia', *Cancer* 19, 1966, 1635–38.

7. J. Schottlaender & F. Kermauner cited in Petersen, 'Precancerous changes …'

8. G.H. Green, 'The treatment of preinvasive carcinoma', lecture notes, 1957. R.W. Jones papers.

9. G. van S. Smith & F.A. Pemberton, 'The picture of very early carcinoma of the uterine cervix', *Surgical Gynecology and Obstetrics* 59, 1934, 1–8.

10. P.A. Younge, A.T. Hertig & A. Armstrong, 'A study of 145 cases of carcinoma *in-situ* of the uterine cervix at the Free Hospital for Women', *American Journal of Obstetrics and Gynecology* 58, 1949, 867–99; P.A. Younge, 'The natural history of carcinoma in-situ of the cervix uteri', *Journal of Obstetrics and Gynaecology of the British Commonwealth* 72, 1965, 9–12.

11. O. Petersen, 'Spontaneous course of cervical precancerous conditions', *American Journal of Obstetrics and Gynecology* 72, 1956, 1063–74.

12. G.N. Papanicoloau and H.F. Traut's classic monograph was *The Diagnosis of Uterine Cancer by the Vaginal Smear* (New York: The Commonwealth Fund, 1943). This was preceded by Papanicoloau and Traut, 'The diagnostic value of vaginal smears in carcinoma of the uterus', *American Journal of Obstetrics and Gynecology* 42, 1941, 193.

13. L. Tasca, A.G. Östör & V. Babes, 'History of gynecologic pathology. XII. Aurel Babeş', *International Journal of Gynecologic Pathology* 21, 2002, 198–202; L.G. Koss, 'A quarter of a century of cytology', *Acta Cytologica* 21, 1977, 639–42.

14. G.L. Wied, 'Pap-test or Babes' method?', Editorial, *Acta Cytologica* 8, 1964, 173–74.

15. L.G. Koss, communication with the author, 18 October 2005.

16. D.A. Boyes, H.K. Fidler & D.R. Lock, 'Significance of *in-situ* carcinoma of the uterine cervix', *British Medical Journal* 5273, 1962, 203–05.

17. D.C. Skegg, P.A. Corwin, C. Paul & R. Doll, 'Importance of the male factor in cancer of the cervix', *Lancet* 320 (8298), 1982, 581–83.

18. R.A. Reynolds & E.M. Temsey (eds), 'History of cervical cancer and the role of the human papilloma virus, 1960–2000', Witness Seminar held by the Wellcome Trust Centre for the History of Medicine at UCL, London, 13 May 2008.

19. E.G. Knox, 'Cervical cytology: A scrutiny of the evidence', in G. McLachlan (ed.), *Problems and Progress in Medical Care* (second series) (London: Nuffield Provincial Hospitals Trust/Oxford University Press, 1966), 279–307.

20. M. Hakama, 'Trends in the incidence of cervical cancer in the Nordic countries', in K. Magnus (ed.), *Trends in Cancer Incidence: Causes and practical implications* (New York: Hemisphere, 1982), 279–92.

21. R. Doll, correspondence with H. McLaren, 1978. In the author's possession.

22. E. Läärä, N. Day & M. Hakama, 'Trends in mortality from cervical cancer in the Nordic countries: Association with organised screening programmes', *Lancet* 1 (8544), 30 May 1987, 1247–49.

23. Fédération Internationale de Gynécologie et d'Obstétrique, Annual Report on the Results of Radiotherapy in Carcinoma of the Uterine Cervix, 1951.

24. A.T. Hertig, P.A. Younge & J.L. McKelvey, 'Debate: What is cancer in-situ of the cervix? Is it the preinvasive form of the true carcinoma?' *American Journal of Obstetrics and Gynecology* 64, 1952, 807–32.

25. J.E. Ayre & C.H. Davis, 'Carcinoma *in-situ*', Correspondence, *Journal of the American Medical Association* 149 (17), 1952, 1594.

26. S. Cartwright, *The Report of the Committee of Inquiry into Allegations Concerning the Treatment of Cervical Cancer at National Women's Hospital and into Other Related Matters* (Auckland: Government Printing Office, 1988), 34.

27. L.G. Koss, F.W. Stewart, F.W. Foote, M.J. Jordan, G.M. Balder & E. Day, 'Some histological aspects of behaviour of epidermoid carcinoma *in-situ* and related lesions of the uterine cervix', *Cancer* 16, 1963, 1160–211.

28. W.A. McIndoe, M.R. McLean, R.W. Jones & P.R. Mullins, 'The invasive potential of carcinoma *in-situ* of the cervix', *Obstetrics and Gynaecology* 64, 1984, 451–58.

29. A.G. Östör, 'The natural history of cervical intraepithelial neoplasia: A critical review', *International Journal of Gynecological Pathology* 12, 1993, 186–92; D.A. Boyes, B. Morrison, E.G. Knox, G.J. Draper & A.B. Miller, 'A cohort study of cervical cancer screening in British Columbia', *Clinical and Investigative Medicine* 5, 1982, 1–29.

30. J.D. Wheeler & A.D. Hertig, 'Carcinoma of the cervix', *American Journal of Clinical Pathology* 25, 1955, 345–72.

31. J. Harbutt, 'New concepts in the treatment of carcinoma of the cervix', *New Zealand Medical Journal* 54, 1955, 356–70.

32. Cartwright, *The Report of the Committee of Inquiry ...*, 34.

33. W.A. McIndoe. In the author's possession.

34. G.H. Green, 'Cervical cancer and cytology screening', *Modern Medicine of New Zealand*, 16 August 1976, 43–46.

35. D. Medley, communication with the author, 2011.

36. J.J. Sullivan in 'Symposium on cervical lesions', *Acta Cytologica* 6, 206, 1962, 191.

37. H.M. Carey & S.E. Williams, 'Cytological diagnosis of preclinical carcinoma *in-situ* of the cervix', *New Zealand Medical Journal* 57, 1958, 227–35.

38. 'Microscopic clues saved lives of 40 women', *New Zealand Herald*, 6 May 1958.

39. G.H. Green, Transcript of Public Hearings to the Committee of Inquiry ...,
   Archives New Zealand BAGC 18494 A638/186 and 187.
40. J.S. Kreiger & L.G. McCormack, 'The indications for conservative therapy for
   intraepithelial carcinoma of the uterine cervix', *American Journal of Obstetrics
   and Gynecology* 76, 1958, 312–20.
41. Cartwright, *The Report of the Committee of Inquiry*, 34.
42. G.H. Green, 'Carcinoma *in-situ* of the uterine cervix: Conservative
   management in 84 of 190 cases', *Australia and New Zealand Journal of
   Obstetrics and Gynaecology* 2, 1962, 49–57.
43. M. McCredie, C. Paul, K. Sharples, J. Baremyai, G. Medley, D.C. Skegg &
   R.W. Jones, 'Consequences in participating in a study of the natural history
   of cervical intraepithelial neoplasia 3', *Australia and New Zealand Journal of
   Obstetrics and Gynaecology* 50, 2010, 363–70.
44. G.H. Green, 'The treatment of preinvasive carcinoma', lecture notes, 1957. In
   the author's possession.
45. G.H. Green, 'Conservative versus radical treatment of carcinoma *in-situ* of
   the uterine cervix', lecture notes, April 1959. In the author's possession.
46. Green, 'Carcinoma *in-situ* of the uterine cervix: Conservative management
   ...'
47. Kreiger & McCormack, 'The indications for conservative therapy ...'
48. 'Cancer testing plan suggested', *New Zealand Herald*, 22 April 1959.
49. 'Female cases cured of cancer seen early', *Auckland Star*, 21 April 1959.
50. W.A. McIndoe, 'A cervical cytology screening programme in the Thames
   area', *New Zealand Medical Journal* 63, 1964, 6–13; W.A. McIndoe, 'Second
   and third years of the study', *New Zealand Medical Journal* 65, 1966, 647–51.
51. M. Coppleson, E. Pixley & B. Reid, *Colposcopy: A scientific and practical
   approach to the cervix in health and disease* (Illinois: Charles C. Thomas,
   1971), fig. 60, 81.
52. M. Coppleson, communication with the author, 2012.
53. Cartwright, *The Report of the Committee of Inquiry*, 34.
54. Annual reports of the National Women's Hospital Post Graduate School of
   Obstetrics and Gynaecology, 1965, 1966, 1967.
55. M. Churchouse, 'The Greening of cytology' (unpublished), 25 May 2010. In
   the author's possession.
56. Coppleson, Pixley & Reid, *Colposcopy*.
57. E. Pixley, 'Basic morphology of the prepubertal and youthful cervix:
   Topographic and hystologic features', *Journal of Reproductive Medicine* 16,
   1976, 221–30.
58. Annual report of the National Women's Hospital Post Graduate School of
   Obstetrics and Gynaecology, 1968.

59. Cartwright, *The Report of the Committee of Inquiry*, 34.
60. G.H. Green, 'Cervical carcinoma *in-situ*: True cancer or non-invasive lesion?', *Australia and New Zealand Journal of Obstetrics and Gynaecology* 4, 1964, 165–73.
61. Annual report of the National Women's Hospital Post Graduate School of Obstetrics and Gynaecology, 1965.
62. G.H. Green, 'The significance of cervical carcinoma *in-situ*', *Australia and New Zealand Journal of Obstetrics and Gynaecology* 6, 1966, 42–44; J.A. Kirkland, 'The cytological and histological diagnosis of dysplasia, carcinoma *in-situ* and early invasive cancer of the cervix', *Australia and New Zealand Journal of Obstetrics and Gynaecology* 6, 1966, 15–19; J.A. Kirkland, 'Chromosomal and mitotic abnormalities in preinvasive and invasive carcinoma of the cervix', *Australia and New Zealand Journal of Obstetrics and Gynaecology* 6, 1966, 35–39.
63. M. Stanley, communication with the author, 29 October 2011.
64. A. Singer, communication with the author, 4 November 2011.
65. Reynolds & Temsey, 'History of cervical cancer and the role of the human papilloma virus', 55.
66. A.W. Liley, 'Intrauterine transfusion of fetus in haemolytic disease', *British Medical Journal* 5365, 2 November 1963, 1107–09.
67. D. Robb, *Medical Odyssey* (Auckland: Collins, 1967), 19.
68. K. Hill, communication with the author, 2012.

CHAPTER 3: AN UNNECESSARY EXPERIMENT

1. J. Stallworthy & G. Bourne, *Recent Advances in Obstetrics and Gynaecology* (London: J. & A. Churchill, 1966), 341.
2. B.F. Heslop, 'All about research: Looking back at the 1987 Cervical Cancer Inquiry', *New Zealand Medical Journal* 117 (1199), 2004.
3. Cartwright, *The Report of the Committee of Inquiry* ..., 21.
4. W.A. McIndoe. In the author's possession.
5. J. Harbutt, communication with the author, 14 February 1995.
6. Cartwright, *The Report of the Committee of Inquiry* ..., 71; W.A. McIndoe, 14 June 1971. In the author's possession.
7. Cartwright, *The Report of the Committee of Inquiry* ..., 21.
8. J.J. Sullivan, Discussion, 'Symposium on cervical lesions', *Acta Cytologica* 6, 1962, 191.
9. G.H. Green, 'Invasive potentiality of cervical carcinoma *in-situ*', *International Journal of Gynecology and Obstetrics* 7, 1969, 157–71.
10. Cartwright, *The Report of the Committee of Inquiry* ..., 21.
11. Ibid., 71.

12. Cartwright, *The Report of the Committee of Inquiry* ..., 70–71.
13. Ibid., 22.
14. G.C. Liggins, communication with B.F. Heslop, 2003. In the author's possession.
15. Minutes of National Women's Hospital Medical Committee, 6 June 1966.
16. Cartwright, *The Report of the Committee of Inquiry* ..., 22.
17. Ibid., 72
18. 'An unfortunate fallout', *Weekend Herald*, 19 September 2009, B2.
19. G.H. Green, 'Cervical carcinoma in-situ', lecture notes, 1968, University of Auckland.
20. Cartwright, *The Report of the Committee of Inquiry* ..., 21.
21. Green. 'Invasive potentiality of invasive carcinoma in-situ'.
22. J. Jordan, 2 August 2001. In the author's possession.

CHAPTER 4: EXPRESSIONS OF CONCERN

1. G.H. Green, 'Cervical carcinoma *in-situ*: True cancer or non-invasive lesion?', *Australia and New Zealand Journal of Obstetrics and Gynaecology* 4, 1964, 165–73.
2. R.W. Jones, personal papers.
3. G.H. Green, 'The significance of cervical carcinoma *in-situ*', *American Journal of Obstetrics and Gynecology* 94, 1966, 1009–22.
4. G.H. Green, 'Is cervical carcinoma *in-situ* a significant lesion?', *International Surgery* 47, 1967, 511–17.
5. G.H. Green, 'Invasive potentiality of invasive carcinoma *in-situ*', *International Journal of Gynecology and Obstetrics* 7, 1969, 157–71.
6. Ibid.; Cartwright, *The Report of the Committee of Inquiry* ..., 78.
7. W.A. McIndoe. In the author's possession.
8. J. Sloane & M. Churchouse, communication with the author.
9. W.A. McIndoe. In the author's possession.
10. Cartwright, *The Report of the Committee of Inquiry* ..., 51; W.A. McIndoe. In the author's possession.
11. M. Churchouse, 'The Greening of cytology', (unpublished) 25 May 2010. In the author's possession.
12. B. Trenwith, communication with the author, 2012.
13. Green, 'Invasive potentiality of invasive carcinoma *in-situ*'.
14. R.W. Jones, personal papers.
15. Ibid.
16. G.H. Green & J.W. Donovan, 'The natural history of carcinoma *in-situ*', *British Journal of Obstetrics and Gynaecology* 77, 1970, 1–9.
17. R.W. Jones, Transcript of Public Hearings to the Committee of Inquiry

..., Archives New Zealand BAGC 18494 A638/186/a. R.W. Jones, personal papers.

18. Green, 'Cervical carcinoma *in-situ*'.

19. W.A. McIndoe. In the author's possession.

20. Green, 'Cervical carcinoma *in-situ*'.

21. J.P. Greenhill, *The Year Book of Obstetrics and Gynecology 1970* (Chicago: Year Book Medical Publishers, 1970), 518–19.

22. M.J. Jordan, in 'Forum: Has the survival rate from invasive carcinoma of the cervix been influenced by cervical screening?', *Modern Medicine USA*, 20 September 1971, 180–88.

23. D.A. Boyes, H.K. Fidler & D.R. Lock, 'Significance of *in-situ* carcinoma of the uterine cervix', *British Medical Journal* 5273, 1962, 203–05.

24. G.H. Green, 'Cervical cancer and cytology screening in New Zealand', *British Journal of Obstetrics and Gynaecology* 85, 1978, 881–86.

25. R.W. Jones, personal papers.

26. J. Jordan, 20 August 2001. In the author's possession.

27. Ibid; J. Murphy, 16 January 2002. In the author's possession.

28. D.F. Hawkins, 16 September 2005. In the author's possession.

29. M. Churchouse, 'The Greening of cytology'.

30. 'NZH cancer smear test "overrated"', *New Zealand Herald*, 27 January 1970; 'Smear test "not reliable"', *New Zealand Herald*, 29 June 1972; 'CIS not a forerunner of invasive cancer', *Auckland Star*, 21 June 1972.

31. W.A. McIndoe. In the author's possession.

32. W.A. McIndoe & S.E. Williams, 'The value of cytology', Correspondence, *New Zealand Medical Journal* 76, 1972, 129.

33. J.F. Giesen, 'The value of cytology', Correspondence, *New Zealand Medical Journal* 76, 1972, 294; G.H. Green, 'Cervical cytology', Correspondence, *New Zealand Medical Journal* 76, 1972, 449–50; J.F. Giesen, 'Cervical cytology', Correspondence, *New Zealand Medical Journal* 77, 1973, 124.

34. I.D. Ronayne, Letter to Senior Medical Staff, 1972; Minutes of National Women's Hospital Senior Medical Staff Committee meeting, 1972. McIndoe papers, in the author's possession.

35. J. Stewart, communication with the author, 2010.

36. S.E. Williams, Letter to G. Wied, 1971. In the author's possession.

37. A. Clarke, *New Zealand Herald*, 4 July 1978.

38. Mee Ling Yeong, communication with the author, December 2014.

39. G.H. Green, 'Cervical cancer in New Zealand: A failure of cytology?', *Asia and Oceania Journal of Obstetrics and Gynaecology* 7, 1981, 303–13.

40. G.R. Duncan, 'Cervical cytology in 1980: Its place and value', *New Zealand Medical Journal* 93, 1981, 119–22.

41. J. Adams, *Cervical Screening Programmes: A review of the literature and its implication for New Zealand* (Wellington: Department of Health, 1991).

42. G. Johannesson & N.E. Day, Correspondence, *British Journal of Obstetrics and Gynaecology* 86, 1979, 671–72.

43. W.A. McIndoe. In the author's possession.

44. R.W. Jones, personal papers.

45. J. Cumming and G. McGuire, communication with the author, 2013.

46. B. Trenwith, communication with the author.

47. P. Herdson. In the author's possession.

48. Ailsa McLean, communication with the author.

49. M.R. McLean, letter to Hospital Medical Committee, 1971.

50. Ailsa McLean, communication with the author.

CHAPTER 5: WHITEWASH

1. G.C. Liggins, Submission to the Committee of Inquiry under Section 13(3) of the Hospitals Act 1957, to inquire into and report on chemotherapy and immunotherapy at Auckland Hospital, 19 April 1974.

2. Dunn to Brych, 21 April 1973. In the author's possession.

3. Ibid.

4. Transcript of evidence to the above inquiry, 9E to 9J4.

5. Editorial, 'A cancer affair', *New Zealand Medical Journal* 80, 1974, 67; 'Report of the Medical Council: Case against Milan Brych', *New Zealand Medical Journal* 85, 1977, 387–90.

6. D. Wright, Report of the Committee of Inquiry under Section 13(3) of the Hospitals Act 1957, to inquire into and report on chemotherapy and immunotherapy at Auckland Hospital, *New Zealand Medical Journal* 80, 1974, 68–71.

7. J. Buchanan, communication with the author, 2012.

8. I. Fisher, communication with the author, 28 February 2005.

9. R. Laurie, communication with the author, 2013.

10. G. Richards, communication with the author, 2010.

11. P. Kolstad, 'Diagnosis and management of precancerous lesions of the cervix uteri', *International Journal of Gynecology and Obstetrics* 4, 1970, 551–60.

12. W.A. McIndoe. In the author's possession.

13. P. Kolstad, correspondence with W. McIndoe, 30 October 1973. In the author's possession.

14. W.A. McIndoe. In the author's possession.

15. M. Davy, communication with the author, 14 November 2012.

16. W.A. McIndoe, memorandum to Medical Superintendent, 10 October 1973. In the author's possession.

17. M.R. McLean, memorandum to Medical Superintendent, 18 October 1973. In the author's possession.
18. G.H. Green, response to McLean's memorandum, 7 November 1973. In the author's possession.
19. Ibid.
20. W.A. McIndoe, memorandum to Medical Superintendent, 14 December 1973. In the author's possession.
21. R.W. Jones, personal papers.
22. M.R. McLean, memorandum to Medical Superintendent, 10 May 1974. In the author's possession.
23. G.H. Green, response to McLean's memorandum, 7 November 1973. In the author's possession.
24. Cartwright, *The Report of the Committee of Inquiry ...*, 76.
25. Ibid., 83.
26. Ibid., 86.
27. Ibid., 88.
28. G.H. Green, 'The progression of preinvasive lesions of the cervix to invasion', *New Zealand Medical Journal* 80, 1974, 279–87.
29. W.A. McIndoe. In the author's possession.
30. R. Doll, 'Concluding remarks', Medical Research Council Epidemiology Symposium, November 1973, *New Zealand Medical Journal* 80, 1974, 403–04.
31. R.W. Jones, personal papers.
32. B. Baguley. In the author's possession.
33. G.H. Green, 'Duration of symptoms and survival rates for invasive cervical cancer', *New Zealand Medical Journal* 10, 1970, 238–43; I. MacDonald, 'Biological predeterminism in human cancer', *Surgery, Gynecology and Obstetrics* 92, 1951, 443–52.
34. B. Baguley. In the author's possession.
35. G.H. Green, 'Duration of symptoms and survival rates for invasive cervical cancer', *Australia and New Zealand Journal of Obstetrics and Gynaecology* 10, 1970, 238; G.H. Green, 'Cancer, dental caries, and radioactive decay: Some aspects of the dental problem', *New Zealand Medical Journal* 79, 1974, 869–73.
36. Green, 'Cancer, dental caries, and radioactive decay'.
37. G.H. Green, Abstract No 69, Proceedings of Otago Medical School Centenary, February 1975.
38. MacDonald, 'Biological predeterminism in human cancer'.
39. National Women's Hospital Postgraduate School Silver Jubilee Meeting Programme, 1976.
40. Green, 'The progression of preinvasive lesions of the cervix to invasion'.
41. W.A. McIndoe, Abstract, 'The invasive potential of carcinoma in situ of the

cervix', *Obstetrical and Gynecological Survey* 34, 1979, 873. In the author's possession.

CHAPTER 6: PHOEBE'S STORY

1. This history has been abstracted from the patient's medical records.
2. T.L.T. Lewis, *Progress in Obstetrics and Gynaecology* (London: J. & A. Churchill, 1956), 558.

CHAPTER 7: NINETEEN EIGHTY-FOUR

1. W.A. McIndoe, 'The invasive potential of carcinoma in situ of the cervix [abstract]', *Obstetrical & Gynecological Survey* 34, 1979, 873; W.A. McIndoe, Presentation to the IFCPC 1978. In the author's possession.
2. J. Jordan, communication with the author.
3. B. Hill, communication with the author, February 2014.
4. M. Churchouse, 'The Greening of cytology'.
5. G. van S. Smith & F.A. Pemberton, 'The picture of very early carcinoma of the uterine cervix', *Surgical Gynecology and Obstetrics* 59, 1934, 1–8; P.A. Younge, A.T. Hertig & A. Armstrong, 'A study of 145 cases of carcinoma *in-situ* of the uterine cervix at the Free Hospital for Women', *American Journal of Obstetrics and Gynecology* 58, 1949, 867–99; O. Petersen, 'Precancerous changes of the cervical epithelium in relation to manifest cervical cancer', *Acta Radiologica*, supplement 127, 1955; Cartwright, *The Report of the Committee of Inquiry* ..., 23.
6. R.W. Jones, 'A medical journal editor's role in exposing an unethical research study', *Obstetrics and Gynecology* 113, January 2009, 161–65.
7. McIndoe, 'The invasive potential of carcinoma in situ of the cervix [abstract]'; McIndoe, Presentation to the IFCPC 1978.
8. This and all following Mattingly quotes are from Jones, 'A medical journal editor's role'.
9. G.H. Green, 'The progression of preinvasive lesions of the cervix to invasion', *New Zealand Medical Journal*, 80, October 1974, 279–87.
10. W.A. McIndoe, 'Cytology or colposcopy', *Australian and New Zealand Journal of Obstetrics & Gynaecology* 8, 1968, 117–18; W.A. McIndoe & G.H. Green, 'Vaginal carcinoma in situ following hysterectomy', *Acta Cytologica* 13, 1969, 158–62; W.A. McIndoe, 'A cervical cytology screening programme in the Thames area', *New Zealand Medical Journal* 63, 1964, 6–13; W.A. McIndoe, 'A cervical screening programme in the Thames area', *New Zealand Medical Journal* 65, 1966, 647–51; W.A. McIndoe & M.J. Churchouse, 'Herpes simplex of the lower genital tract in the female', *Australia and New Zealand Journal of Obstetrics and Gynaecology* 12, 1972, 14–23.

11. Jones, 'A medical journal editor's role'.
12. Ibid.
13. Cartwright, *The Report of the Committee of Inquiry ...*, 92.
14. A.B. MacLean, communication with the author, 1981.
15. Cartwright, *The Report of the Committee of Inquiry ...*, 92.
16. R.W. Jones, W.A. McIndoe & M.R. McLean, 'The invasive potential of carcinoma *in-situ* of the cervix', in S. Kurihara, K. Noda, Y. Tenjin, H. Kubo & T. Kasamatsu (eds), 'Cervical pathology and colposopy. Proceedings of the Fifth World Congress of the International Federation for Cervical Pathology and Colposcopy, Tokyo, Japan', *Excerpta Medica,* Amsterdam, 1985.
17. Jones, 'A medical journal editor's role'.
18. Unnamed referee's report for *Obstetrics and Gynecology*. In the author's possession.
19. Jones, 'A medical journal editor's role'.
20. W.A. McIndoe, M.R. McLean, R.W. Jones & P.R. Mullins, 'The invasive potential of carcinoma *in-situ* of the cervix', *Obstetrics and Gynaecology,* Vol. 64, October 1984, 451–58.
21. Ibid.
22. Ibid.; P. Kolstad and O. Klem, 'Long term follow-up of 1121 cases of carcinoma in situ', *Obstetrics and Gynecology* 48, 1976, 125.
23. C. Wall, 'The glamorous gynaecologists at National Women's Hospital', *Metro,* June 1984, 36, 32–50.

CHAPTER 8: ANNUS HORRIBILIS

1. D.C. Skegg, C. Paul, R.J. Seddon, N.W. Fitzgerald et al, 'Recommendations for routine cervical screening', *New Zealand Medical Journal* 98, 1985, 636–39.
2. G.R. Duncan, T.C. Svensen & R.W. Jones, 'Screening for cervical cancer', Correspondence, *New Zealand Medical Journal* 98, 1985, 821.
3. G.H. Green, 'Screening for cervical cancer', Correspondence, *New Zealand Medical Journal* 98, 1985, 968.
4. D.C. Skegg, 'Cervical screening', Correspondence, *New Zealand Medical Journal* 99, 1986, 26–27.
5. P. Skrabanek & M. Jamieson, 'Eaten by worms: A comment on cervical cancer screening', *New Zealand Medical Journal* 98, 1985, 654.
6. Anna Storey, 'Cancer rates dropping slowly', *Auckland Star,* 5 October 1986; Linda Dyson, 'Testing times', *More,* March 1987, 119.
7. D.G. Bonham, G.H. Green & G.C. Liggins, 'Cervical human papilloma virus infection and colposcopy', *Australia and New Zealand Medical Journal of Obstetrics and Gynaecology* 27, 1987, 131.
8. S. Coney, *The Unfortunate Experiment: The full story behind the inquiry into cervical cancer treatment* (Auckland: Penguin Books, 1998), 33.

9. M.A.H. Baird, communication with the author, 24 May 2010.

10. Coney, *The Unfortunate Experiment*, 15.

11. P. Kolstad and O. Klem, 'Long term follow-up of 1121 cases of carcinoma in situ', *Obstetrics and Gynecology* 48, 1976, 125.

12. Coney, *The Unfortunate Experiment*, 24.

13. J. McAuliffe, communication with the author, 9 April 1985.

14. Coney, *The Unfortunate Experiment*, 18.

15. Ibid., 25.

16. C. Matheson, *Fate Cries Enough: A survivor of the cervical cancer experiment at National Women's Hospital* (Auckland: Sceptre, 1989), 64.

17. Ibid., 83.

18. Coney, *The Unfortunate Experiment*, 40.

19. M. Whaley, communication with the author, 2014.

20. Coney, *The Unfortunate Experiment*, 47.

21. R.W. Jones, Proceedings of the 4th World Congress of the International Federation of Cervical Pathology and Colposcopy, 1981.

22. R.W. Jones & M.R. McLean, 'Carcinoma *in-situ* of the vulva: A review of 31 treated and 5 untreated cases', *Obstetrics and Gynecology* 68, 1986, 499–503.

CHAPTER 9: IRRECONCILABLE DIFFERENCES

1. S. Coney & P. Bunkle, An unfortunate experiment at National Women's, *Metro*, June 1987, 46–65.

2. J. Corbett, 'Second thoughts on the unfortunate experiment', *Metro*, July 1990, 54–73.

3. S. Coney, *The Unfortunate Experiment: The full story behind the inquiry into cervical cancer treatment* (Auckland: Penguin Books, 1998), 71.

4. Ibid.

5. Minutes of the Auckland Hospital Board Finance and General Purposes Committee, 8 June 1987.

6. Anonymous. Correspondence with Dr A.L. Honeyman, 30 October 1986 and 7 November 1986.

7. S. Cartwright, *The Report of the Committee of Inquiry into Allegations Concerning the Treatment of Cervical Cancer at National Women's Hospital and into Other Related Matters* (Auckland: Government Printing Office, 1988).

8. 'Woman judge for Cervical Cancer Inquiry', *Evening Post*, 10 June 1987.

9. Coney, *The Unfortunate Experiment*, 79; 'Inquiry will clear Green', *Evening Post*, 11 June 1982.

10. M. Churchouse, communication with the author, August 2014.

11. Minutes of the Auckland Hospital Board Finance and General Purposes Committee, 30 November 1987.

12. Ibid., P. Davis, tabled statement.
13. 'Who will monitor the doctors?', *Sunday Star*, 7 July 1987; 'Cancer doctor: No guinea pigs, my conscience is clear', *New Zealand Herald*, 11 June 1987; Coney, *The Unfortunate Experiment*, 78.
14. M.R. McLean, communication with the author.
15. H. Rennie, communication with the author.
16. 'Jockeying for position', *Auckland Star*, 23 October 1987.
17. Cartwright, personal papers, National Archives.
18. Theresa Gattung, 'When the music stops', *North & South*, April 2013.
19. Ibid.
20. G.H. Green, Transcript of Public Hearings to the Committee of Inquiry ..., Archives New Zealand BAGC 18494 A638/186/a.
21. Ibid.
22. G.H. Green, Report to University of Auckland following sabbatical leave, 1980.
23. B.F. Heslop, personal papers; Coney, *The Unfortunate Experiment*.
24. G.H. Green, Transcript of Public Hearings to the Committee of Inquiry ...,
25. Ibid.
26. Ibid.
27. '"Questions misled me" says Green', *Auckland Sun*, 8 September 1987.
28. Cartwright, *The Report to the Committee of Inquiry ...*, 33.
29. 'Dr Green "one of the first feminists"', *New Zealand Herald*, 10 November 1987; C. Mantell, 'Inquiry told: Dr Green gave hope', *New Zealand Herald*, 28 October 1987; 'Some are calling me a murderer', *Auckland Sun*, 3 September 1987.
30. G.H. Green, Transcript of Public Hearings to the Committee of Inquiry ...,
31. Green v Attorney-General, HC Wellington CP560/87 [1987] NZHC 324 (5 November 1987).
32. D.G. Bonham, Transcript of Public Hearings to the Committee of Inquiry ..., Archives New Zealand BAGC 18494 A638/189/190/a.
33. Ibid.
34. Ibid.
35. Ibid.
36. M.A.H. Baird, Transcript of Public Hearings to the Committee of Inquiry ..., Archives New Zealand BAGC18494 A638/191/a.
37. B. Faris, Transcript of Public Hearings to the Committee of Inquiry ..., Archives New Zealand BAGC18494 A638/191/a.
38. E. Pixley, communication with the author, 10 September 1987.
39. E. Pixley, Transcript of Public Hearings to the Committee of Inquiry ..., Archives New Zealand BAGC18494 A638/188/a.

40. Noda and Ueki, Transcript of Public Hearings to the Committee of Inquiry …, Archives New Zealand BAGC18494 A638/189/a.

41. Jamieson and Macintosh, Transcript of Public Hearings to the Committee of Inquiry …, Archives New Zealand BAGC18494 A638/197/a.

42. Cartwright, *The Report of the Committee of Inquiry* …, 58.

43. Ibid., 105.

44. R.M. Richart, Transcript of Public Hearings to the Committee of Inquiry …, Archives New Zealand BAGC18494 A638/186/a.

45. R.W. Jones, personal papers. J. Jordan, communication with the author.

46. J. Jordan, Transcript of Public Hearings to the Committee of Inquiry …, Archives New Zealand BAGC18494 A638/188/a.

47. P. Kolstad, Transcript of Public Hearings to the Committee of Inquiry …, Archives New Zealand BAGC18494 A638/199/a.

48. M. Coppleson, Evidence of Dr Malcolm Coppleson, Sydney, 19 December 1987, before Judge Cartwright with Counsel assisting Ms Goddard and Commission advisor Dr Charlotte Paul. In the author's possession.

49. D.G. Skegg, Transcript of Public Hearings to the Committee of Inquiry …, Archives New Zealand BAGC18494 A638/193/a.

50. Ibid.

51. Cartwright, *The Report of the Committee of Inquiry* …, 141.

52. 'Question out of perspective', *Dominion*, 12 November 1987.

53. Cartwright, *The Report of the Committee of Inquiry* …, 141.

54. R.W. Jones, Transcript of Public Hearings to the Committee of Inquiry …, Archives New Zealand BAGC18494 A638/197/a.

55. Ibid.

56. R.W. Jones, personal research, unpublished.

57. G.H. Green, 'Cervical carcinoma *in-situ.* An atypical viewpoint', *Australia and New Zealand Journal of Obstetrics and Gynaecology* 10, 1970, 41–48.

58. M. Vennell, Transcript of Public Hearings to the Committee of Inquiry …, Archives New Zealand BAGC18494 A638/194/a.

59. Correspondence, Rodney Harrison to Counsel Assisting Cervical Cancer Inquiry, 21 December 1987.

60. Meeting between Judge Cartwright and Margaret Vennell, 4 February 1988, Side Issues raised during the Inquiry, Archives New Zealand BAGC18491 A638/192/a.

61. S. Cartwright, correspondence with Vice Chancellor, University of Auckland, 2 March 1988.

62. 'Doctors too powerful, witness tells inquiry', *New Zealand Herald*, 10 December 1989; M. O'Regan, Transcript of Public Hearings to the Committee of Inquiry …, Archives New Zealand BAGC18494 A638/198/a.

63. Cartwright, *The Report of the Committee of Inquiry ...*, 75.
64. Ibid., 60.
65. Ibid.

CHAPTER 10: AFTERMATH

1. S. Coney, 'The end of the experiment', *New Zealand Listener*, 10 September 1988.
2. M.A.H. Baird, Correspondence, *New Zealand Listener*, 29 October 1988.
3. Minutes of the National Women's Hospital Medical Committee, 8 August 1988.
4. Minutes of the National Women's Hospital Medical Committee, 15 September 1988.
5. Minutes of the National Women's Hospital Medical Committee, 22 September 1988.
6. M.A.H. Baird, Letter to Medical Superintendent, 10 September 1988.
7. Royal New Zealand College of Obstetricians and Gynaecologists, Newsletter No. 2, 1988; Minutes of Extraordinary General Meeting, Wellington, 23 September 1988.
8. Ronayne, presentation to Extraordinary General Meeting of the Royal New Zealand College of Obstetricians and Gynaecologists, Wellington, 23 September 1988.
9. Ibid.
10. Ibid.
11. M.A.H. Baird, correspondence with Professor R. Seddon, 13 September 1988.
12. Minutes of the Annual General Meeting of the Royal New Zealand College of Obstetricians and Gynaecologists, Auckland, 11 August 1989.
13. S. Coney, *The Unfortunate Experiment: The full story behind the inquiry into cervical cancer treatment* (Auckland: Penguin Books, 1998).
14. Royal New Zealand College of Obstetricians and Gynaecologists, Newsletter No. 2, 1988; Minutes of Extraordinary General Meeting, Wellington, 23 September 1988.
15. Minutes of the meeting of Combined Medical Staff, Greenlane/National Women's Hospitals, 14 September 1990.
16. Ibid.
17. R. Hilliker, 'Cancer docs face changes', *Sunday Star Times*, 4 February 1990.
18. Correspondence, Women's Health Council to Dr Alexander, Chairman of the Medical Council of New Zealand, 27 February 1990.
19. C. Wall, 'The new feminism', *Metro*, July 1984.
20. G. Arthur, NZ Medical Association newsletter, January 1989.
21. M.A.H. Baird, NZ Medical Association newsletter, February 1989.

22. Minutes of NZ Medical Association Council, 10 August 1988. Quoted by Klim McPherson, *New Zealand Medical Journal* 102, 1989, 169.
23. Coney, 'The end of the experiment', 25.
24. L. Taylor, Correspondence, *New Zealand Listener*, 8 October 1988.
25. 'Cartwright Report based on a scam', *Dominion Sunday Times*, 12 March 1989.
26. Minutes of Auckland Division of Specialists in Obstetrics and Gynaecology, 5 July 1990.
27. J. Corbett, 'Second thoughts on the unfortunate experiment at National Women's', *Metro*, July 1990, 54–73.
28. W. Roger, Editorial, 'My town: Intellectual thuggery', *Metro*, September 1990.
29. Corbett, 'Second thoughts on the unfortunate experiment'.
30. R.W. Jones, Correspondence, 'A guerrilla campaign?', *Metro*, October 1990, 17–18.
31. M.A.H. Baird, Opinion, *Metro*, September 1990.
32. E. Geiringer, 'The triumph of victimocracy', *Metro*, October 1990, 134.
33. H. Clark, Ministerial Statement, 23 September 1990.
34. 'Doctor does not know best', Editorial, *Auckland Star*, 14 March 1989.
35. S. Cartwright, *The Report of the Committee of Inquiry into Allegations Concerning the Treatment of Cervical Cancer at National Women's Hospital and into Other Related Matters* (Auckland: Government Printing Office, 1988), 101.
36. S. Coney, Correspondence, '26 deaths can be confirmed', *Sunday Star Times*, 27 May 1990; M.A.H. Baird, Correspondence, 'Death numbers', *Sunday Star Times*, 1 July 1990.
37. 'Doubts about wisdom of mass screening', *Auckland Star*, 21 June 1972.
38. B. Cox, communication with the author, 30 August 2012.
39. Coney, *The Unfortunate Experiment*, 270.
40. Ibid., 271.
41. Review of Recent Criticism of the Report of the Cervical Cancer Inquiry 1988 by the Public Issues Committee of the Auckland District Law Society, 18 October 1990.
42. R.W. Jones, 'Reflections on carcinoma in situ', *New Zealand Medical Journal* 104, August 1991, 339–41.

CHAPTER 11: RIGHT OR WRONG: HEAL OR HARM

1. Kevin Mitchell, 'All's fair (and always has been) in sport', *Observer*, London, 13 November 1994, 27.
2. Anonymous, 'The delineation of internal organs by an electrical method', *British Medical Journal* 2 (2909), 1916, 459–61.

3. Letter from Geoffrey Chamberlain, Royal College of Obstetricians and Gynaecologists, London, 28 November 1994. In the author's possession.

4. *British Medical Journal*, 309, 1994, 1459.

5. Ibid.

6. Letter from Royal College of Obstetricians and Gynaecologists, London, 7 December 1994.

7. M.J. Churchouse, G.N. Carter & D.G. Bonham, 'The source of 6-phosphogluconate dehydrogenase in vaginal fluid samples', *Journal of Obstetrics and Gynaecology British Commonwealth* 74, 1967, 712–22.

8. M.J. Churchouse, communication with the author, August 2014.

9. S. Lock & F. Wells, *Fraud and Misconduct in Medical Research* (London: British Medical Journal Publishing Group, 1993), IX.

10. R. Dresser, 'Defining scientific misconduct', *Journal of the American Medical Association* 269, 1993, 895–97.

11. N. Wade, Book review, *New England Journal of Medicine* 328, 1993, 1648–49.

12. Dresser, 'Defining scientific misconduct'.

13. B. Macfarlane, *Researching with Integrity: The ethics of academic inquiry* (New York and London: Routledge, 2009).

14. J. Colquhoun, cited in Macfarlane, *Researching with Integrity*, 56–57.

15. L. Fesinger, *A Theory of Cognitive Dissonance* (Stanford: Stanford University Press, 1957).

16. W. Weyers, *The Abuse of Man* (New York: Ardor Scribendi, 2003), 356–60.

17. Ibid., 493–502.

18. G.H. Green, 'Invasive potentiality of invasive carcinoma in-situ', *International Journal of Gynecology and Obstetrics* 7, 1969, 157–71; Annual Report of the National Women's Hospital Postgraduate School of Obstetrics and Gynaecology, 1966.

19. J.C. Fletcher, 'A case study in historical relativism: The Tuskegee (Public Health Service) Syphilis Study', in Susan M. Revervy (ed.), *Tuskegee Truths: Rethinking the Tuskegee Syphilis Study* (Chapel Hill: University of North Carolina Press, 2000), 276–98.

20. A. Koestler, *The Case of the Midwife Toad* (London: Hutchinson, 1971).

21. J. Hixon, *A Patchwork Mouse* (Garden City, NY: Anchor Press–Doubleday, 1976).

22. British Medical Association (New Zealand Branch), *Annual Handbook*, 1965–1966, 14–19.

23. Weyers, *The Abuse of Man*, 567.

24. H.K. Beecher, 'Ethics and clinical research', *New England Journal of Medicine*, 274, June 1966, 367–73.

25. Weyers, *The Abuse of Man*, 382–84.

26. Ibid., 573.

27. M.H. Pappworth, *Human Guinea Pigs: Experimentation on man* (London: Routledge & Kegan Paul, 1967); M.H. Pappworth, obituary, *British Medical Journal* 309, 1994, 1577.

28. G.H. Green, 'Tubal ligation', *New Zealand Medical Journal* 57, 1958, 470–77.

29. C. Quin, personal papers.

30. P.B. Sim, 'The legal duty to warn patients of risk in treatment', *New Zealand Medical Journal* 64, 1965, 250–52.

31. Ibid.

32. Hospitals Amendment Act 1957, Archives New Zealand, BAGC A638 18494.

33. M.A.H. Baird, Correspondence, *New Zealand Medical Journal* 118, 2005.

34. S. Cartwright, draft memorandum, 'The appointment of the committee', n.d., National Archives.

35. Cartwright, *The Report of the Committee of Inquiry ...*, 153–57.

36. R. Farrell, V. Gebski & N.F. Hacker, 'Quality of life after complete lymphadenectomy for vulvar cancer: Do women prefer sentinel lymph node biopsy?', *International Journal of Gynecological Cancer* 24 (4), 2014, 813–19.

37. Cartwight, *The Report of the Committee of Inquiry ...*, 127.

38. E. Friedson, *Profession of Medicine* (New York: Dodd, 1975).

39. N. Hacker, Interview for *Medical Observer*, 1990.

40. At another cancer inquiry Professor Donald Evans of the Bioethics Centre at Otago University incorrectly stated in evidence that we would have been able to do the research for our 1984 paper because we were the clinicians responsible for the cases. Of course most of the cases in question were Green's. Report of the Ministerial Inquiry into the Under-reporting of Cervical Smear Abnormalities in the Gisborne Region, April 2001.

41. J. Hopkins, 'Life after Cartwright', *New Zealand Medical Journal* 102 (862), 1989, 71.

42. B.F. Heslop & A.J. Gray, Correspondence, 'Medical research: Who minds the minders?', *New Zealand Medical Journal* 102, 1989, 141.

43. E.J. Rossiter, 'Reflections of a whistle-blower', *Nature* 357 (6378), 11 June 1992, 434–36.

CHAPTER 12: MABEL'S STORY

1. All quotes in this chapter are from the records of the Australian doctor, including copies of letters from Green and the pathologists, radiotherapists and other gynaecologists involved.

CHAPTER 13: A PROFESSION DIVIDED

1. Frank Rutter: http://nationalwomenshealth.adhb.govt.nz/about-us/our-history/1970-1980

2.   M. Hambly, communication with the author.
3.   A. Gray, correspondence, *New Zealand Medical Journal* 103, August 1990, 378.
4.   C. Wright Mills, *The Power Elite* (New York: Oxford University Press, 1956), 3–4.
5.   University of Auckland, Report of the University Council Sub-committee on the Cartwright Report, 9 February 1989.
6.   J.R. Hampton, 'The end of clinical freedom', *British Medical Journal* 287, 1983, 1237–38.
7.   D. Owen, *In Sickness and in Power* (London: Methuen, 2008).
8.   W.A. McIndoe. In the author's possession.
9.   Cartwright, *The Report of the Committee of Inquiry ...*, 22.
10. J.C. Fletcher, 'A case study in historical relativism', *Journal of the National Medical Association* 87, 1995, 56–67.
11. Gray, Correspondence, *New Zealand Medical Journal* 103, August 1990, 378.
12. M. Scott, Report of the New Zealand Conference on Women and Health, organised by the Committee on Women and the Department of Health, 1977.
13. Ibid.
14. Ibid.
15. B.F. Heslop, personal papers. In the author's possession.
16. S. Coney, *The Unfortunate Experiment: The full story behind the inquiry into cervical cancer treatment* (Auckland: Penguin Books, 1998), 75.
17. Ibid., 40.
18. Pat Rosier, 'The speculum bites back: Feminists spark an inquiry into the treatment of carcinoma in-situ at Auckland's National Women's Hospital', *Reproductive and Genetic Engineering* 2, 1989, 121–32.
19. Editorial, 'The lessons from the Savage Inquiry', *British Medical Journal* 290, 1985, 285–86.
20. Ibid.
21. G.H. Green, 'The progression of preinvasive lesions of the cervix to invasion', *New Zealand Medical Journal* 80, 1974, 279–87.
22. Ibid.
23. L.G. Koss, communication with the author, 18 October 2005.
24. A.B. Miller, correspondence and communication with the author, 12 May 2001.
25. E.G. Knox, 'Cervical cytology: A scrutiny of the evidence', in G. McLachlan (ed.), *Problems and Progress in Medical Care* (2nd series) (London: Nuffield Provincial Hospitals Trust/Oxford University Press, 1966), 279–307.
26. L. Wright, personal communication with the author.
27. Anonymous, medical friend of Green.
28. L. Schellekens, communication with the author.

CHAPTER 14: MEA CULPA

1. D.G. Bonham, G.H. Green & G.C. Liggins, 'Cervical human papilloma virus infection and colposcopy', *Australia and New Zealand Journal of Obstetrics and Gynaecology* 27, 1987, 131.
2. Anonymous, medical friend of Green.
3. B.F. Heslop, personal papers. In the author's possession.
4. B.F. Heslop, '"All about research": Looking back at the 1987 Cervical Cancer Inquiry', *New Zealand Medical Journal* 117, August 2004.
5. B.F. Heslop, personal papers. In the author's possession.
6. Angus McIndoe, communication with the author, 29 April 2011.
7. I.D. Ronayne, communication with the author.
8. B.F. Heslop, personal papers, letter dated 28 December 2011. In the author's possession.
9. M. Henaghan, *Health Professionals and Trust: The cure for healthcare law & policy* (Abingdon: Routledge Cavendish, 2011).
10. K. McPherson, Correspondence, *New Zealand Medical Journal* 102, 1989, 169.
11. A.C. Baier, *Moral Prejudices: Essays on ethics* (Cambridge, Massachusetts: Harvard University Press, 1984).
12. C. Paul, 'Internal and external morality of medicine: Lessons from New Zealand', *British Medical Journal*, 2000, 499–503.
13. Ibid.
14. F. Lewin, *Bioethics for Health Professionals: An introduction and critical approach* (South Yarra, Australia: Palgrave McMillan, 1996).
15. P. Ball, *Serving the Reich: The struggle for the soul of physics under Hitler* (London: Vintage Books, 2013).
16. M. Taylor, 'Science is enforced humility', *Guardian Weekly*, 13 November 2012.
17. B. Kyle, communication with the author.
18. C. Quin, personal papers.
19. Cartwright, *The Report of the Committee of Inquiry …*, 265–67.
20. Ibid.
21. S. Coney, 'Take the power from the docs', *Broadsheet*, July/August 1989.

EPILOGUE

1. 'It was wrong says Bonham', *Sunday Star Times*, 9 December 1990.

POSTSCRIPT

1. Minutes of National Women's Senior Medical Officers meeting, 20 August 2009.

2. L. Bryder, *A History of the 'Unfortunate Experiment' at National Women's Hospital* (Auckand: Auckland University Press, 2009).

3. J. Manning (ed.), Introduction, *The Cartwright Papers: Essays on the Cervical Cancer Inquiry 1987–88* (Wellington: Bridget Williams Books, 2009), 19.

4. B. Brookes, 'The making of a controversy', in J. Manning (ed.), *The Cartwright Papers: Essays on the Cervical Cancer Inquiry 1987–88* (Wellington: Bridget Williams Books, 2009), 102.

5. C. Paul, 'The cervical cancer study', in J. Manning (ed.), *The Cartwright Papers: Essays on the Cervical Cancer Inquiry 1987–88* (Wellington: Bridget Williams Books, 2009), 138.

6. Ibid., 118; C. Mantell, 'Cancer scandal', Correspondence, *New Zealand Listener*, 29 September 2009; M.A.H. Baird, 'Cancer scandal', Correspondence, *New Zealand Listener*, 5 September 2009.

7. Dan O'Connor. Personal papers in the author's possession.

8. 'An unfortunate fallout', *Weekend Herald*, 19 September 2009, B2.

9. C. Paul & B. Brookes, 'The rationalization of unethical research: Revisionist accounts of the Tuskagee Syphillus Study and the New Zealand "Unfortunate Experiment"', *American Journal of Public Health* 105, 2015; M.A. Baird et al., Correspondence, *American Journal of Public Health* 106, 2016.

10. I.C. Chalmers, communication with the author, 17–24 February 2014.

11. L. Bryder, *TV One News*, 14 February 2014.

12. R.W. Jones, 'Why did so many develop cancer?', *New Zealand Medical Journal*, 30 July 2010, 123: www.nzma.org.nz/journal/123-1319/4245/; R.W. Jones, 'Historians and patients', Correspondence, *New Zealand Listener*, 19 April 2014.

13. B.F. Heslop, personal papers. In possession of author.

14. I. Chalmers, communication with the author, 20 February 2014.

15. M.R. McCredie, C. Paul, K.J. Sharples, J. Baranyai, G. Medley, D.C. Skegg & R.W. Jones, 'Consequences in participating in a study of the natural history of cervical intraepithelial neoplasia 3', *Australia and New Zealand Journal of Obstetrics and Gynaecology* 50, 2010, 363–70.

16. R.W. Carrell, 'Trial by media', *Notes and Records of the Royal Society* 66 (3), 2012, 301–06.

17. Ellie Mae O'Hagan, 'Feminists can be sexy and funny – but it's anger that changes the world': www.theguardian.com/commentisfree/2013/feb/26/feminists-sexy-funny-anger-changes-world

BIBLIOGRAPHY

OFFICIAL REPORTS AND DOCUMENTS

Adequacy of Medical Statistics in New Zealand, report of ad hoc committee of Medical Research Council of New Zealand, November 1969.

Annual reports of the National Women's Hospital Post Graduate School of Obstetrics and Gynaecology, 1965, 1966, 1967, 1968.

Bonham, D.G., Affidavit to Medical Council, 1990, 22.

Butler, N.R. & Bonham, D.G., *Perinatal Mortality: The first report of the 1958 British Perinatal Mortality Survey under the auspices of National Birthday Trust Fund* (London: E. & S. Livingstone, 1963).

Cartwright, S., *The Report of the Committee of Inquiry into Allegations Concerning the Treatment of Cervical Cancer at National Women's Hospital and into Other Related Matters* (Auckland: Government Printing Office, 1988).

Liggins, G.C., Submission to the Committee of Inquiry under Section 13(3) of the Hospitals Act 1957, to inquire into and report on chemotherapy and immunotherapy at Auckland Hospital, 19 April 1974.

Fédération Internationale de Gynécologie et d'Obstétrique, Annual Report on the Results of Radiotherapy in Carcinoma of the Uterine Cervix, 1951.

Green, G.H., Report to University of Auckland following sabbatical leave, 1980.

Green v Attorney-General, HC Wellington CP560/87 [1987] NZHC 324 (5 November 1987).

Report of the Ministerial Inquiry into the Under-reporting of Cervical Smear Abnormalities in the Gisborne Region, April 2001.

Scott, M., Report of the New Zealand Conference on Women and Health, organised by the Committee on Women and the Department of Health, 1977.

Transcript of Public Hearings to the Committee of Inquiry into Allegations Concerning the Treatment of Cervical Cancer at National Women's Hospital and into Other Related Matters, Archives New Zealand BAGC 18494 A638/186, 186/a, 187, 188/a, 189/a, 190/a, 191/a, 192/a, 193/a, 194/a, 197/a, 198/a, 199/a

University of Auckland Council Papers, 1963.

University of Auckland, Report of the University Council Sub-committee on the Cartwright Report, 9 February 1989.

Wright, D., Report of the Committee of Inquiry under Section 13(3) of the Hospitals Act 1957, to inquire into and report on chemotherapy and immunotherapy at Auckland Hospital, *New Zealand Medical Journal* 80, 1974, 68–71.

MINUTES

Minutes of the Annual General Meeting of the Royal New Zealand College of Obstetricians and Gynaecologists, Auckland, 11 August 1989.

Minutes of Auckland Division of Specialists in Obstetrics and Gynaecology, 5 July 1990.

Minutes of Auckland Hospital Board Finance and General Purposes Committee, 8 June 1987; 30 November 1987.

Minutes of the meeting of Combined Medical Staff, Greenlane/National Women's Hospitals, 14 September 1990.

Minutes of National Women's Hospital Medical Committee, 6 June 1966; 18 August, 15 September, 22 September 1988.

Minutes of National Women's Hospital Senior Medical Staff Committee, 1972.

Minutes of National Women's Senior Medical Officers, 20 August 2009.

Minutes of NZ Medical Association Council, 10 August 1988.

Minutes of NZ Obstetric and Gynaecological Society, vol. 1, 11 December 1940, 196.

Minutes of Royal New Zealand College of Obstetricians and Gynaecologists, Extraordinary General Meeting, Wellington, 23 September 1988.

JOURNAL, MAGAZINE AND NEWSPAPER ARTICLES

'An unfortunate fallout', Weekend Herald, 19 September 2009, B2.

'An unfortunate fallout: Academics against revisionist history', New Zealand Herald, 19 September 2009.

Anonymous, 'The delineation of internal organs by an electrical method', British Medical Journal 2 (2909), 1916, 459–61.

Ayre, J.E. & Davis, C.H., 'Carcinoma in-situ', Correspondence, Journal of the American Medical Association 149 (17), 1952, 1594.

Baird, M.A.H., 'Cancer scandal', Correspondence, New Zealand Listener, 5 September 2009.

Baird, M.A.H. et al., Correspondence, American Journal of Public Health 106, 2016, 1208–10.

Beecher, H.K., 'Ethics and clinical research', New England Journal of Medicine, 274, June 1966, 367–73.

Bonham, D.G. & Gibb, D.F., 'A new enzyme test for gynaecological cancer', British Medical Journal 2 (5308), 1962, 823–44.

Bonham, D.G., Green, G.H. & Liggins, G.C., 'Cervical human papilloma virus infection and colposcopy', Australia and New Zealand Medical Journal of Obstetrics and Gynaecology 27, 1987, 131.

Boyes, D.A., Fidler, H.K. & Lock, D.R., 'Significance of in-situ carcinoma of the uterine cervix', British Medical Journal 5273, 1962, 203–05.

Boyes, D.A., Morrison, B., Knox, E.G., Draper, G.J. & Miller, A.B., 'A cohort study of cervical cancer screening in British Columbia', *Clinical and Investigative Medicine* 5, 1982, 1–29.

Broders, A.C., 'Carcinoma *in-situ* contrasted with benign penetrating epithelium', *Journal of the American Medical Association* 99, 1932, 1670–74.

British Medical Journal, 309, 1994, 1459

'Cancer doctor: No guinea pigs, my conscience is clear', *New Zealand Herald*, 11 June 1987.

'Cancer testing plan suggested', *New Zealand Herald*, 22 April 1959.

Carey, H.M. & Williams, S.E., 'Cytological diagnosis of preclinical carcinoma *in-situ* of the cervix', *New Zealand Medical Journal* 57, 1958, 227–35.

Carrell, R.W., 'Trial by media', *Notes and Records of the Royal Society* 66 (3), 2012, 301–06.

'Cartwright Report based on a scam', *Dominion Sunday Times*, 12 March 1989.

Churchouse, M.J., Carter G.N. & Bonham, D.G., 'The source of 6-phosphogluconate dehydrogenase in vaginal fluid samples', *Journal of Obstetrics Gynaecology British Commonwealth* 74, 1967, 712–22.

'CIS not a forerunner of invasive cancer', *Auckland Star*, 21 June 1972.

Clarke, A., *New Zealand Herald*, 4 July 1978.

Coney, S., 'The end of the experiment', *New Zealand Listener*, 10 September 1988.

_____, *Broadsheet*, July/August 1989.

_____, Correspondence, '26 deaths can be confirmed', *Sunday Star Times*, 27 May 1990.

Coney, S. & Bunkle, P., 'An unfortunate experiment at National Women's', *Metro*, June 1987, 46–65.

Corbett, J., 'Second thoughts on the unfortunate experiment', *Metro*, July 1990, 54–73.

'DES not the villain, says doctor', *Auckland Star*, 28 August 1981.

'Doctor does not know best', Editorial, *Auckland Star*, 14 March 1989.

'Doctors too powerful, witness tells inquiry', *New Zealand Herald*, 10 December 1989.

Doll, R., 'Concluding remarks', Medical Research Council Epidemiology Symposium, November 1973, *New Zealand Medical Journal* 80, 1974, 403–04.

'Doubts about wisdom of mass screening', *Auckland Star*, 21 June 1972.

'Dr Green "one of the first feminists"', *New Zealand Herald*, 10 November 1987.

Dresser, R., 'Defining scientific misconduct', *Journal of the American Medical Association* 269, 1993, 895–97.

Duncan, G.R., 'Cervical cytology in 1980: Its place and value', *New Zealand Medical Journal* 93, 1981, 119–22.

Duncan, G.R., Svensen, T.C. & Jones, R.W., 'Screening for cervical cancer', Correspondence, *New Zealand Medical Journal* 98, 1985, 821.

Dyson, L., 'Testing times', *More*, March 1987, 119.

Editorial, 'A cancer affair', *New Zealand Medical Journal* 80, 1974, 67.

Editorial, 'The lessons from the Savage Inquiry', *British Medical Journal* 290, 1985, 285–86.

'Female cases cured of cancer seen early', *Auckland Star*, 21 April 1959.

Farrell, R., Gebski, V. & Hacker, N.F., 'Quality of life after complete lymphadenectomy for vulvar cancer: Do women prefer sentinel lymph node biopsy?', *International Journal of Gynecological Cancer* 24 (4), 2014, 813–19.

Fletcher, J.C., 'A case study in historical relativism', *Journal of the National Medical Association* 87, 1995, 56–67.

'Forum: Has the survival rate from invasive carcinoma of the cervix been influenced by cervical screening?', *Modern Medicine USA*, 20 September 1971, 180–88.

Gattung, T., 'When the music stops', *North & South*, April 2013

Geiringer, E., 'The triumph of victimocracy', *Metro*, October 1990, 134.

Giesen, J.F., 'The value of cytology', Correspondence, *New Zealand Medical Journal* 76, 1972, 294.

————,'Cervical cytology', Correspondence, *New Zealand Medical Journal* 77, 1973, 124.

Gray, A., correspondence, *New Zealand Medical Journal* 103, August 1990, 378.

Green, G.H., 'Tubal ligation', *New Zealand Medical Journal* 57, 1958, 470–77.

————, 'Carcinoma *in-situ* of the uterine cervix: Conservative management in 84 of 190 cases', *Australia and New Zealand Journal of Obstetrics and Gynaecology* 2, 1962, 49–57.

————, 'Letter from New Zealand: New York horizons', *Bulletin of the Sloane Hospital for Women* 9, Winter 1963, 133–36.

————, 'Cervical carcinoma *in-situ*: True cancer or non-invasive lesion?', *Australia and New Zealand Journal of Obstetrics and Gynaecology* 4, 1964, 165–73.

————, 'The significance of cervical carcinoma *in-situ*', *Australia and New Zealand Journal of Obstetrics and Gynaecology* 6, 1966, 42–44.

————, 'The significance of cervical carcinoma *in-situ*', *American Journal of Obstetrics and Gynecology* 94, 1966, 1009–22.

————, 'Is cervical carcinoma *in-situ* a significant lesion?', *International Surgery* 47, 1967, 511–17.

————, 'A royal obstetric tragedy and the epitaph', *NZ Nursing Journal*, July 1969, 7–11.

————, 'Invasive potentiality of cervical carcinoma *in-situ*, *International Journal of Gynecology and Obstetrics* 7, 1969, 157–71.

————, 'Cervical carcinoma *in-situ*: An atypical viewpoint', *Australia and New Zealand Journal of Obstetrics and Gynaecology* 10, 1970, 41–48.

_____, 'Duration of symptoms and survival rates for invasive cervical cancer', *Australia and New Zealand Journal of Obstetrics and Gynaecology* 10, 1970, 238.

_____, 'Cervical cytology', Correspondence, *New Zealand Medical Journal* 76, 1972, 449–50.

_____, 'Cancer, dental caries, and radioactive decay: Some aspects of the dental problem', *New Zealand Medical Journal* 79, 1974, 869–73.

_____, 'The progression of preinvasive lesions of the cervix to invasion', *New Zealand Medical Journal* 80, 1974, 279–87.

_____, Abstract No 69, Proceedings of Otago Medical School Centenary, February 1975.

_____, 'Cervical cancer and cytology screening', *Modern Medicine of New Zealand*, 16 August 1976, 43–46.

_____, 'Cervical cancer and cytology screening in New Zealand', *British Journal of Obstetrics and Gynaecology* 85, 1978, 881–86.

_____, 'Cervical cancer in New Zealand: A failure of cytology?', *Asia and Oceania Journal of Obstetrics and Gynaecology* 7, 1981, 303–13.

_____, 'A Tudor caesarean section', *Surgery, Gynecology and Obstetrics* 161, 1985, 490–96.

_____, 'Screening for cervical cancer', Correspondence, *New Zealand Medical Journal* 98, 1985, 968.

Green, G.H. & Donovan, J.W., 'The natural history of carcinoma *in-situ*', *British Journal of Obstetrics and Gynaecology* 77, 1970, 1–9.

Hampton, J.R., 'The end of clinical freedom', *British Medical Journal* 287, 1983, 1237–38.

Harbutt, J., 'New concepts in the treatment of carcinoma of the cervix', *New Zealand Medical Journal* 54, 1955, 356–70.

Hertig, A.T., Younge, P.A. & McKelvey, J.L., 'Debate: What is cancer in-situ of the cervix? Is it the preinvasive form of the true carcinoma?' *American Journal of Obstetrics and Gynecology* 64, 1952, 807–32.

Heslop, B.F., 'All about research: Looking back at the 1987 Cervical Cancer Inquiry', *New Zealand Medical Journal* 117 (1199), 2004.

Heslop, B.F. & Gray, A.J., Correspondence, 'Medical research: Who minds the minders?', *New Zealand Medical Journal* 102, 1989, 141.

Hilliker, R., 'Cancer docs face changes', *Sunday Star Times*, 4 February 1990.

Hopkins, J., 'Life after Cartwright', *New Zealand Medical Journal* 102 (862), 1989, 71.

Howie, R.N., 'Credit where credit's due', *New Zealand Herald*, 20 July 2005.

'Inquiry will clear Green', *Evening Post*, 11 June 1982.

'It was wrong says Bonham', *Sunday Star Times*, 9 December 1990.

'Jockeying for position', *Auckland Star*, 23 October 1987.

Johannesson, G. & Day, N.E., Correspondence, *British Journal of Obstetrics and Gynaecology* 86, 1979, 671–72.

Jones, R.W., Correspondence, 'A guerrilla campaign?', *Metro*, October 1990, 17–18.

_____, 'Reflections on carcinoma in situ', *New Zealand Medical Journal* 104, August 1991, 339–41.

_____, 'A medical journal editor's role in exposing an unethical research study', *Obstetrics and Gynecology* 113, January 2009, 161–65.

_____, 'Why did so many develop cancer?', *New Zealand Medical Journal*, 30 July 2010, 123: www.nzma.org.nz/journal/123-1319/4245/

_____, 'Historians and patients', Correspondence, *New Zealand Listener*, 19 April 2014.

Jones, R.W., McIndoe, W.A. & McLean, M.R., 'The invasive potential of carcinoma *in-situ* of the cervix', in S. Kurihara, K. Noda, Y. Tenjin, H. Kubo & T. Kasamatsu (eds), 'Cervical pathology and colposopy. Proceedings of the Fifth World Congress of the International Federation for Cervical Pathology and Colposcopy, Tokyo, Japan', *Excerpta Medica*, Amsterdam, 1985.

Jones, R.W. & McLean, M.R., 'Carcinoma *in-situ* of the vulva: A review of 31 treated and 5 untreated cases', *Obstetrics and Gynecology* 68, 1986, 499–503.

Jordan, M.J, in 'Forum: Has the survival rate from invasive carcinoma of the cervix been influenced by cervical screening?', *Modern Medicine USA*, 20 September 1971, 180–88.

Kirkland, J.A., 'Chromosomal and mitotic abnormalities in preinvasive and invasive carcinoma of the cervix', *Australia and New Zealand Journal of Obstetrics and Gynaecology* 6, 1966, 35–39.

_____, 'The cytological and histological diagnosis of dysplasia, carcinoma *in-situ* and early invasive cancer of the cervix', *Australia and New Zealand Journal of Obstetrics and Gynaecology* 6, 1966, 15–19.

Kolstad, P., 'Diagnosis and management of precancerous lesions of the cervix uteri', *International Journal of Gynecology and Obstetrics* 4, 1970, 551–60.

Koss, L.G., 'A quarter of a century of cytology', *Acta Cytologica* 21, 1977, 639–42.

Koss, L.G., Stewart, F.W., Foote, F.W., Jordan, M.J., Balder, G.M. & Day, E., 'Some histological aspects of behaviour of epidermoid carcinoma *in-situ* and related lesions of the uterine cervix', *Cancer* 16, 1963, 1160–211.

Kreiger, J.S. & McCormack, L.G., 'The indications for conservative therapy for intraepithelial carcinoma of the uterine cervix', *American Journal of Obstetrics and Gynecology* 76, 1958, 312–20.

Läära, E., Day, N. & Hakama, M., 'Trends in mortality from cervical cancer in the Nordic countries: Association with organised screening programmes', *Lancet* 1 (8544), 30 May 1987, 1247–49.

Liggins, G.C., Article marking retirement of G.H. Green, *University of Auckland News* 11, 1981, 31.

Liggins, G.C. & Howie, R.N., 'A controlled trial of antepartum glucocorticoid treatment for prevention of respiratory distress syndrome in premature infants', *Paediatrics* 50, 1972, 515–25.

Liley, A.W., 'Intrauterine transfusion of fetus in haemolytic disease', *British Medical Journal* 5365, 2 November 1963, 1107–09.

Mantell, C., 'Inquiry told: Dr Green gave hope', *New Zealand Herald*, 28 October 1987.

_____, 'Cancer scandal', Correspondence, *New Zealand Listener*, 29 September 2009.

MacDonald, I., 'Biological predeterminism in human cancer', *Surgery, Gynecology and Obstetrics* 92, 1951, 443–52.

McCredie, M.R., Paul, C., Sharples, K., Baranyai, J., Medley, G., Skegg, D.C. & Jones, R.W., 'Consequences in participating in a study of the natural history of cervical intraepithelial neoplasia 3', *Australia and New Zealand Journal of Obstetrics and Gynaecology* 50, 2010, 363–70.

McCredie, M.R., Sharples, K., Paul, C., Baranyai, J., Medley, G., Skegg, D.C. & Jones, R.W., 'Natural history of cervical neoplasia and risk of invasive cancer in women with cervical intraepithelial neoplasia 3: A retrospective cohort study', *Lancet Oncology* 9, 2008, 425–34.

McIndoe, W.A., 'A cervical cytology screening programme in the Thames area', *New Zealand Medical Journal* 63, 1964, 6–13.

_____, 'Second and third years of the study', *New Zealand Medical Journal* 65, 1966, 647–51.

_____, 'Cytology or colposcopy', *Australian and New Zealand Journal of Obstetrics & Gynaecology* 8, 1968, 117–18.

_____, 'The invasive potential of carcinoma in situ of the cervix [abstract]', *Obstetrical & Gynecological Survey* 34, 1979, 873.

McIndoe, W.A. & Churchouse, M.J., 'Herpes simplex of the lower genital tract in the female', *Australia and New Zealand Journal of Obstetrics and Gynaecology* 12, 1972, 14–23.

McIndoe, W.A. & Green, G.H., 'Vaginal carcinoma in situ following hysterectomy', *Acta Cytologica* 13, 1969, 158–62.

McIndoe, W.A., McLean, M.R., Jones, R.W. & Mullins, P.R., 'The invasive potential of carcinoma *in-situ* of the cervix', *Obstetrics and Gynaecology* 64, 1984, 451–58.

McIndoe, W.A. & Williams, S.E., 'The value of cytology', Correspondence, *New Zealand Medical Journal* 76, 1972, 129.

McLaren, H.C., Attwood, M.E., Nixon, W.C., Bonham, D.G., MacRae, D.J., Hawkins D.F. & Eton, B., 'Discussion on the cervix–antepartum and postpartum', *Proceedings of the Royal Society of Medicine* 54, 1961, 712–20.

McPherson, K., Correspondence, *New Zealand Medical Journal* 102, 1989, 169.

'Microscopic clues saved lives of 40 women', *New Zealand Herald*, 6 May 1958.

Mitchell, Kevin, 'All's fair (and always has been) in sport', *Observer*, London, 13 November 1994, 27.

National Health Statistics Centre, 'Perinatal mortality in New Zealand 1972–73', Special Report Series 50 (Wellington: Department of Health, 1977).

'NZH cancer smear test "overrated"', *New Zealand Herald*, 27 January 1970.

Obituary, D.G. Bonham, *University of Auckland News* 35, 2005, 20–21.

Obituary, B.V. Kyle, *New Zealand Medical Journal* 121, 2008, 1269.

Obituary, M.H. Pappworth, *British Medical Journal* 309, 1994, 1577.

Obituary, D. Robb, *New Zealand Medical Journal* 80, 1974, 128–32.

Östör, A.G., 'The natural history of cervical intraepithelial neoplasia: A critical review', *International Journal of Gynecological Pathology* 12, 1993, 186–92.

Paul, C., 'Internal and external morality of medicine: Lessons from New Zealand', *British Medical Journal*, 2000, 499–503.

Paul, C. & Brookes, B., 'The rationalization of unethical research: Revisionist accounts of the Tuskagee Syphillus Study and the New Zealand "Unfortunate Experiment"', *American Journal of Public Health* 105, 2015.

Petersen, O., 'Precancerous changes in the cervical epithelium in relation to manifest cervical cancer', *Acta Radiologica*, supplement 127, 1955.

Pixley, E., 'Basic morphology of the prepubertal and youthful cervix: Topographic and hystologic features', *Journal of Reproductive Medicine* 16, 1976, 221–30.

'Question out of perspective', *Dominion*, 12 November 1987.

'"Questions misled me" says Green', *Auckland Sun*, 8 September 1987.

Reagan, J.W., Seidemann, I.L. & Saracusa, Y., 'The cellular morphology of carcinoma *in-situ* and dysplasia or atypical hyperplasia of the uterine cervix', *Cancer* 6, 1953, 224–35.

'Report of the Medical Council: Case against Milan Brych', *New Zealand Medical Journal* 85, 1977, 387–90.

Reynolds, R.A. & Temsey, E.M. (eds), 'History of cervical cancer and the role of the human papilloma virus, 1960–2000', Witness Seminar held by the Wellcome Trust Centre for the History of Medicine at UCL, London, 13 May 2008.

Richart, R.M., 'Influence of diagnostic and therapeutic procedures on the distribution of cervical intraepithelial neoplasia', *Cancer* 19, 1966, 1635–38.

Roger, W., Editorial, 'My town: Intellectual thuggery', *Metro*, September 1990.

Rosier, P., 'The speculum bites back: Feminists spark an inquiry into the treatment of carcinoma in-situ at Auckland's National Women's Hospital', *Reproductive and Genetic Engineering* 2, 1989, 121–32.

Rossiter, E.J., 'Reflections of a whistle-blower', *Nature* 357 (6378), 11 June 1992, 434–36.

Rubin, I.C., 'The pathological diagnosis of incipient carcinoma of the uterus', *American Journal of Obstetrics and Diseases of Women and Children* 62, 1910, 668–76.

Sim, P.B., 'The legal duty to warn patients of risk in treatment', *New Zealand Medical Journal* 64, 1965, 250–52.

Skegg, D.C., 'Cervical screening', Correspondence, *New Zealand Medical Journal* 99, 1986, 26–27.

Skegg, D.C., Corwin, P.A., Paul, C. & Doll, R., 'Importance of the male factor in cancer of the cervix', *Lancet* 320 (8298), 1982, 581–83.

Skegg, D.C., Paul, C., Seddon, R.J., Fitzgerald, N.W. et al, 'Recommendations for routine cervical screening', *New Zealand Medical Journal* 98, 1985, 636–39.

Skrabanek, P. & Jamieson, M., 'Eaten by worms: A comment on cervical cancer screening', *New Zealand Medical Journal* 98, 1985, 654.

'Smear test "not reliable"', *New Zealand Herald*, 29 June 1972.

Smith, G. van S. & Pemberton, F.A., 'The picture of very early carcinoma of the uterine cervix', *Surgical Gynecology and Obstetrics* 59, 1934, 1–8.

'Some are calling me a murderer', *Auckland Sun*, 3 September 1987.

Storey, A., 'Cancer rates dropping slowly', *Auckland Star*, 5 October 1986.

Sullivan, J.J., Discussion, 'Symposium on cervical lesions', *Acta Cytologica* 6, 206, 1962, 191.

Tasca, L., Östör A.G. & Babes, V., 'History of gynecologic pathology. XII. Aurel Babeş', *International Journal of Gynecologic Pathology* 21, 2002, 198–202.

Taylor, L., Correspondence, *New Zealand Listener*, 8 October 1988.

Taylor, M., 'Science is enforced humility', *Guardian Weekly*, 13 November 2012.

Wade, N., Book review, *New England Journal of Medicine* 328, 1993, 1648–49.

Wall, C., 'The glamorous gynaecologists at National Women's Hospital', *Metro*, June 1984, 36, 32–50.

_____, 'The new feminism', *Metro*, July 1984.

Wheeler, J.D. & Hertig, A.D., 'Carcinoma of the cervix', *American Journal of Clinical Pathology* 25, 1955, 345–72.

'Who will monitor the doctors?', *Sunday Star*, 7 July 1987.

Wied, G.L., 'Pap-test or Babes' method?', Editorial, *Acta Cytologica* 8, 1964, 173–74.

Williams, J., Harveian Lectures for 1886: 'On cancer of the uterus', *Lancet*, 1 January 1887, 6–9; 8 January 1887, 59–62.

'Woman judge for Cervical Cancer Inquiry', *Evening Post*, 10 June 1987.

Wright, D., Report of the Committee of Inquiry under Section 13(3) of the Hospitals Act 1957, to inquire into and report on chemotherapy and immunotherapy at Auckland Hospital, *New Zealand Medical Journal* 80, 1974, 68–71.

Younge, P.A., 'The natural history of carcinoma in-situ of the cervix uteri', *Journal of Obstetrics and Gynaecology of the British Commonwealth* 72, 1965, 9–12.

Younge, P.A., Hertig, A.T. & Armstrong, A., 'A study of 145 cases of carcinoma *in-situ* of the uterine cervix at the Free Hospital for Women', *American Journal of Obstetrics and Gynecology* 58, 1949, 867–99.

BOOKS AND BOOK CHAPTERS

Adams, J., *Cervical Screening Programmes: A review of the literature and its implication for New Zealand* (Wellington: Department of Health, 1991).

Baier, A.C., *Moral Prejudices: Essays on ethics* (Cambridge, Massachusetts: Harvard University Press, 1984).

Ball, P., *Serving the Reich: The struggle for the soul of physics under Hitler* (London: Vintage Books, 2013).

Belgrave, M., *The Mater: A history of Auckland's Mercy Hospital 1900–2000* (Auckland: Mercy Hospital, 2000).

British Medical Association (New Zealand Branch), *Annual Handbook*, 1965–1966.

Brookes, B., 'The making of a controversy', in J. Manning (ed.), *The Cartwright Papers: Essays on the Cervical Cancer Inquiry 1987–88* (Wellington: Bridget Williams Books, 2009).

Butler, N.R. & Bonham, D.G., *Perinatal Mortality: The first report of the 1958 British Perinatal Mortality Survey under the auspices of National Birthday Trust Fund* (London: E. & S. Livingstone, 1963).

Cartwright, S., *The Report of the Committee of Inquiry into Allegations Concerning the Treatment of Cervical Cancer at National Women's Hospital and into Other Related Matters* (Auckland: Government Printing Office, 1988).

Chamberlain, G., *Special Delivery: The life of the celebrated British obstetrician William Nixon* (London: Royal College of Obstetricians and Gynaecologists Press, 2004).

Coney, S., *The Unfortunate Experiment: The full story behind the inquiry into cervical cancer treatment* (Auckland: Penguin Books, 1998).

Coppleson, M., Pixley, E. & Reid, B., *Colposcopy: A scientific and practical approach to the cervix in health and disease* (Illinois: Charles C. Thomas, 1971).

Fesinger, L., *A Theory of Cognitive Dissonance* (Stanford: Stanford University Press, 1957).

Fletcher, J.C., 'A case study in historical relativism: The Tuskegee (Public Health Service) Syphilis Study', in Susan M. Revervy (ed.), *Tuskegee Truths: Rethinking the Tuskegee Syphilis Study* (Chapel Hill: University of North Carolina Press, 2000), 276–98.

Friedson, E., *Profession of Medicine* (New York: Dodd, 1975).

Green, G.H., *Introduction to Obstetrics* (Christchurch: N.M. Peryer, 4 edns, 1962–82).

_____, chapter on the history of the Postgraduate School of Obstetrics and Gynaecology, in H.D. Erlam (ed.), *A Notable Result: An historical essay on the beginnings and first fifteen years of the School of Medicine* (Auckland: University of Auckland School of Medicine, 1983), 68.

Greenhill, J.P., *The Year Book of Obstetrics and Gynecology 1970* (Chicago: Year Book Medical Publishers, 1970).

Hakama, M., 'Trends in the incidence of cervical cancer in the Nordic countries', in K. Magnus (ed.), *Trends in Cancer Incidence: Causes and practical implications* (New York: Hemisphere, 1982), 279–92.

Henaghan, M., *Health Professionals and Trust: The cure for healthcare law & policy* (Abingdon: Routledge Cavendish, 2011).

Hixon, J., *A Patchwork Mouse* (Garden City, NY: Anchor Press–Doubleday, 1976).

Knox, E.G., 'Cervical cytology: A scrutiny of the evidence', in G. McLachlan (ed.), *Problems and Progress in Medical Care* (2nd series) (London: Nuffield Provincial Hospitals Trust/Oxford University Press, 1966), 279–307.

Koestler, A., *The Case of the Midwife Toad* (London: Hutchinson, 1971).

Lewin, F., *Bioethics for Health Professionals: An introduction and critical approach* (South Yarra, Australia: Palgrave McMillan, 1996).

Lewis, T.L.T., *Progress in Obstetrics and Gynaecology* (London: J. & A. Churchill, 1956).

Lock, S., & Wells, F., *Fraud and Misconduct in Medical Research* (London: British Medical Journal Publishing Group, 1993).

Macfarlane, B., *Researching with Integrity: The ethics of academic inquiry* (New York and London: Routledge, 2009).

Manning, J., (ed.), Introduction, *The Cartwright Papers: Essays on the Cervical Cancer Inquiry 1987–88* (Wellington: Bridget Williams Books, 2009), 19.

Matheson, C., *Fate Cries Enough: A survivor of the cervical cancer experiment at National Women's Hospital* (Auckland: Sceptre, 1989).

O'Hagan, Ellie Mae, 'Feminists can be sexy and funny – but it's anger that changes the world': www.theguardian.com/commentisfree/2013/feb/26/feminists-sexy-funny-anger-changes-world

Owen, D., *In Sickness and in Power* (London: Methuen, 2008).

Pappworth, M.H., *Human Guinea Pigs: Experimentation on man* (London: Routledge & Kegan Paul, 1967).

Paul, C., 'The cervical cancer study', in J. Manning (ed.), *The Cartwright Papers: Essays on the Cervical Cancer Inquiry 1987–88* (Wellington: Bridget Williams Books, 2009).

Robb, D., *Medical Odyssey* (Auckland: Collins, 1967).

Sparrow, M., *Abortion Then and Now* (Wellington: Victoria University Press, 2010).

Stallworthy, J. & Bourne, G., *Recent Advances in Obstetrics and Gynaecology* (London: J. & A. Churchill, 1966).

Weyers, W., *The Abuse of Man* (New York: Ardor Scribendi, 2003).

Wright Mills, C., *The Power Elite* (New York: Oxford University Press, 1956).

CORRESPONDENCE WITH AUTHOR

Chalmers, I.C., 17–24 February 2014.

Churchouse, M.J., August 2014.

Cox, B., 30 August 2012.

Hawkins, D.F., 16 September 2005.

McIndoe, A., 29 April 2011.

Miller, A.B., 12 May 2001.

OTHER

Bryder, L., *TV One News*, 14 February 2014.

Hacker, N., Interview for *Medical Observer*, 1990.

New Zealand Medical Association newsletter: January 1989; February 1989.

Review of Recent Criticism of the Report of the Cervical Cancer Inquiry 1988 by the Public Issues Committee of the Auckland District Law Society, 18 October 1990.

Royal New Zealand College of Obstetricians and Gynaecologists, Newsletter No. 2, 1988.

INDEX

Page numbers in roman numerals indicate illustrations.